simply
incredible
MEATS

CREATIVE VEGAN MEAT SOLUTIONS

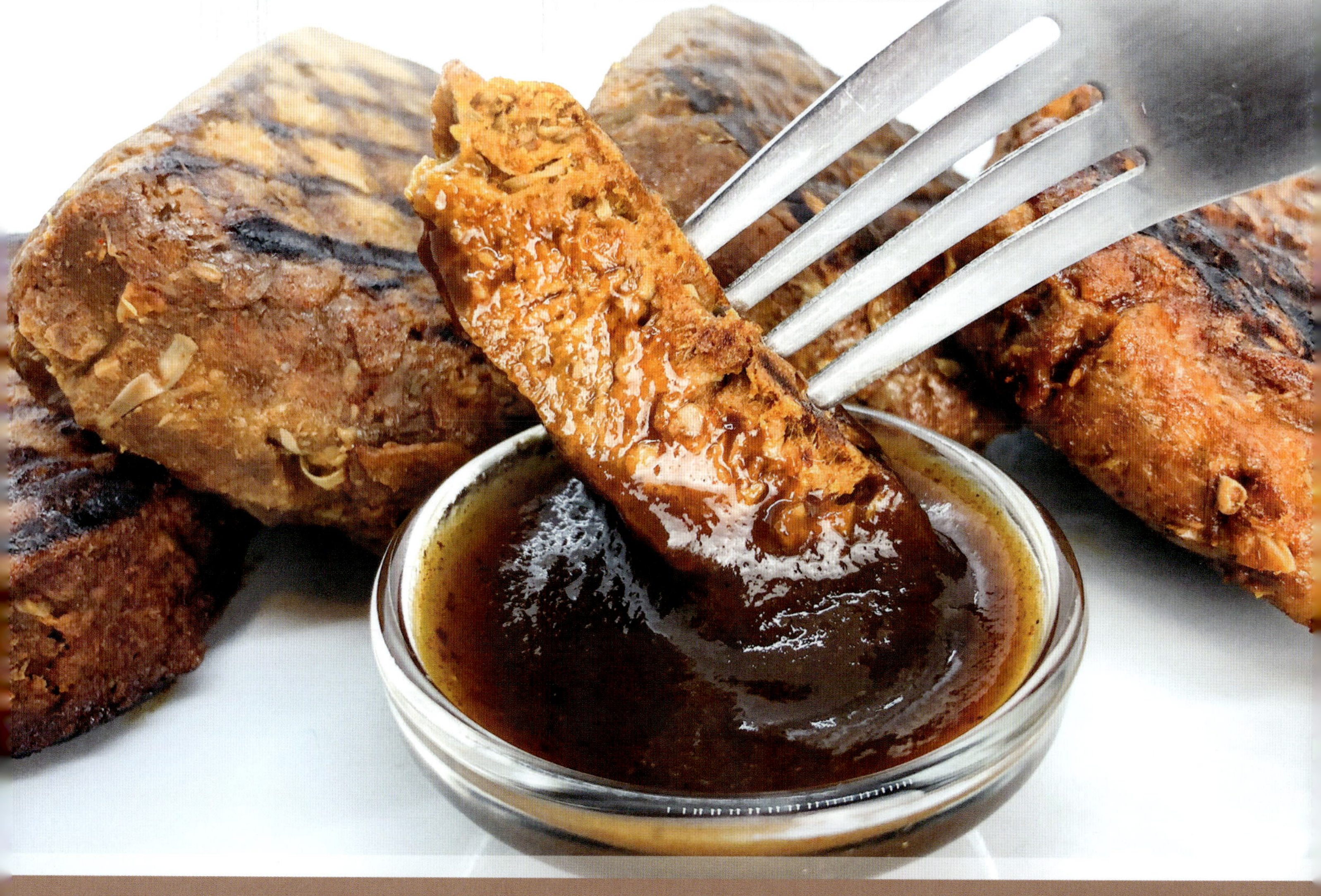

chef mark anthony

SIMPLY INCREDIBLE VEGAN MEAT

ISBN 13: 978-0-9828791-9-1

ISBN 10: 0-9828791-9-9

Layout and cover design: Lanette Steiner

To order books, request information, or comment, please contact:

MARK ANTHONY

Address: Box 6103 . South Bend, IN 46660

Email: tvchefmarkanthony@gmail.com

Printed in the United States of America

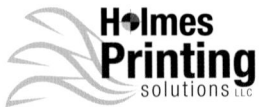

8757 County Road 77 . Fredericksburg, OH 44627 | p. 888.473.6870

INTRODUCTION

Welcome to the world of *Simply Incredible Vegan Meat*. I believe that you are quickly going to realize that these are some of the best vegan meat recipes we have ever produced.

When I first contemplated the thought of developing a book with vegan meats, it was quite overwhelming. But as with any challenge, it all starts with one a single step. So I started to set the parameters. I wanted recipes to meet 5 criteria.

First, it has to look like meat. Second, it has to taste like meat. Third, it has to have the texture of meat. Fourth, and possibly the most critical, it must be far healthier than the real thing. And fifth, it has to be simple enough to not scare away anyone who wants to have fun in the kitchen.

This book has literally been years in the making. Many of the recipes have been tested and tried dozens of times. Sometimes the failure on one recipe would show me a concept that produced success on another recipe.

The recipes in this book so closely resemble a meat counterpart, that some of my vegan friends refused to try them! However, the benefit of incorporating these dishes as a meat replacer, is that they can help many people fill a void that they are missing from their prior meat filled diets. These recipes can literally be a great transition tool, when people are ready to make a switch to a plant based diet. And these recipes are fun!! They are fun to create, fun to share, and fun as a conversation piece next time you invite your friends and family over for lunch. You can literally use this book as a witnessing tool.

I give all the credit to our Heavenly Father who inspired each recipe and provided the energy and motivation to persevere in working through every detail.

Be Healthy, Be Blessed,

Mark Anthony

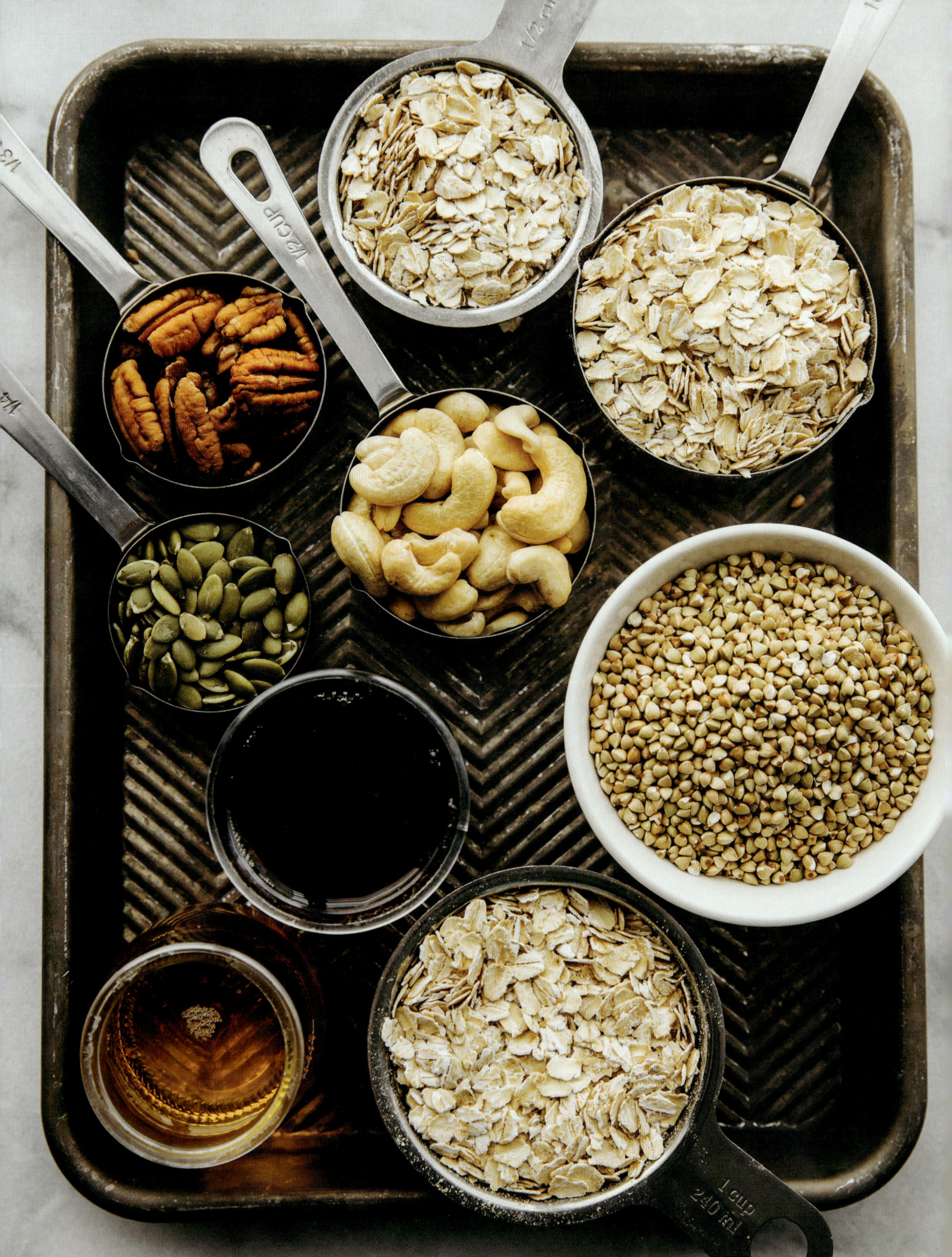

RECIPES

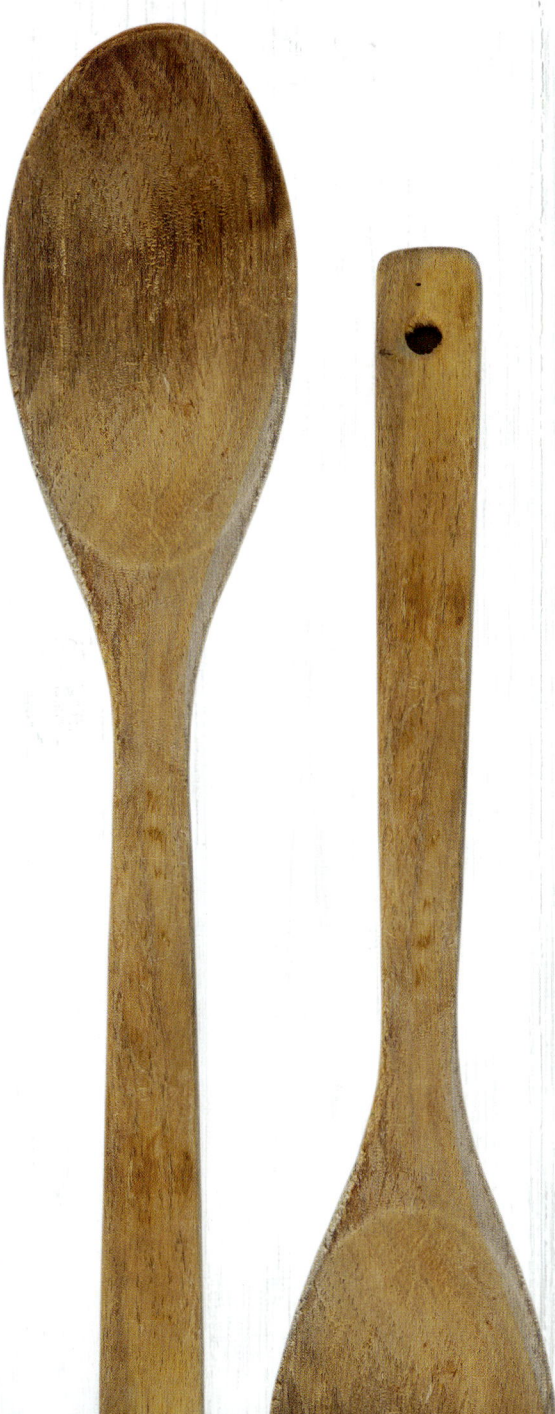

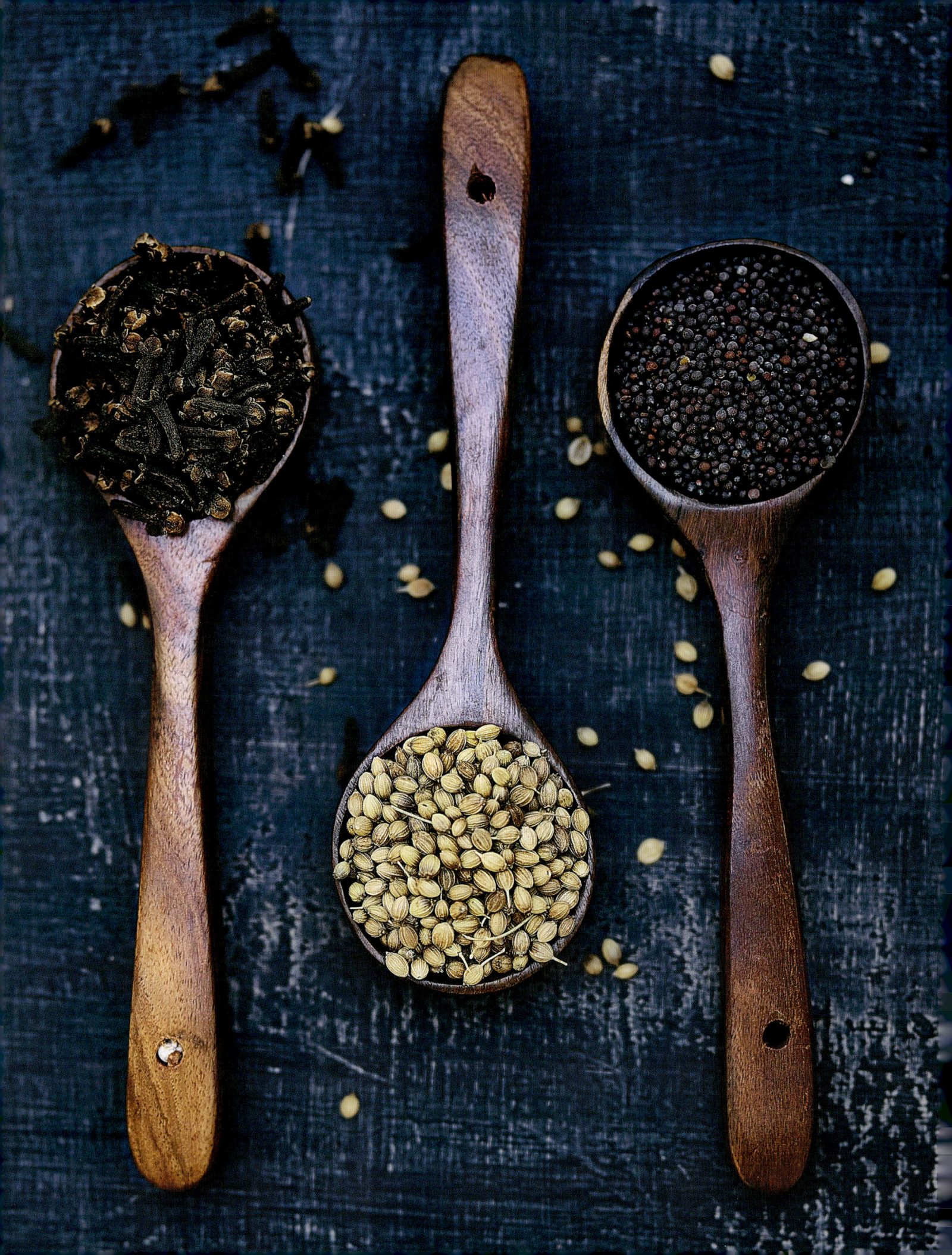

RESOURCES

ALL ABOUT COMMERCIALLY PRODUCED VEGAN MEATS

There are a lot of really good, available vegan meats on store shelves, and there are some to stay away from. The first concern with these products, is the price. You are paying for convenience. Pound for pound, they can be as expensive as real meat. And the sad part is that most of them are made with very inexpensive foods. Why should something that is made with flour and beans be more expensive than say chicken or steak?

Lets focus on some of the good products out there, and how you can recognize the best of the best. Here are some questions to ask when shopping:

DOES THE PRODUCT CONTAIN DAIRY PRODUCTS? Many of the vegetarian meat substitutes are actually made with whey protein, eggs and other dairy products.

WHAT IS THE FAT CONTENT? Many of the store bought products are loaded with fat and have a high caloric content. And it's usually not a good fat.

LOOK AT THE SODIUM CONTENT. Many meat replacement products are loaded with sodium, much more than we should consume.

IS THE PRODUCT MADE WITH GMOS? Yes, they are often made with the non-organic GMO products.

DOES THE PRODUCT HAVE CHEMICALS? There are a lot of new brands of vegan meats that use chemicals to achieve the perfect taste and texture. There are also many, healthy ingredients that you may not recognize. So don't assume that an unusual sounding name is unhealthy.

MY TOP 10 VEGAN MEAT SUBSTITUTES

When you are looking for meat substitutes, you don't always have to go to the extreme like I have in this book. I intended for this book to be fun and creative. But in all reality, I personally enjoy more whole foods in their natural state.

In this section I wanted to share with you a few items in my regular diet that would be my typical substitutes for meat. Many of these I will serve with a minimal amount of prep work or and little no oil. Spices are always used generously to get the variety you need.

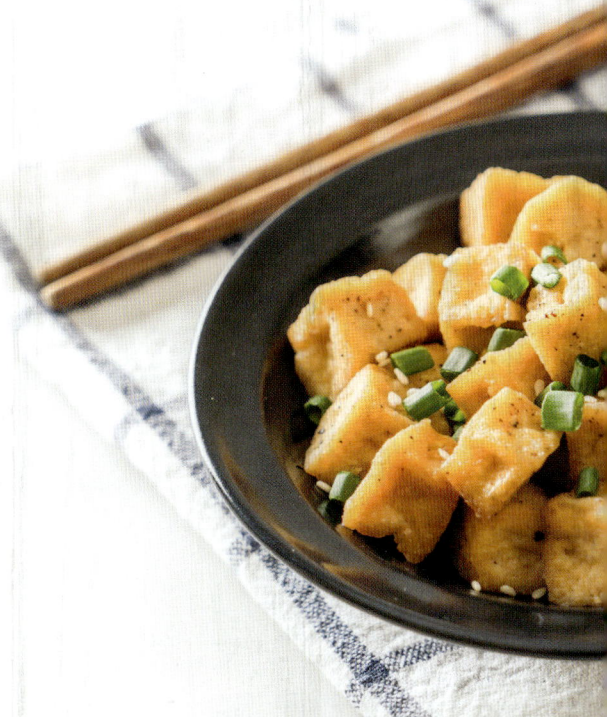

BEANS AND LEGUMES

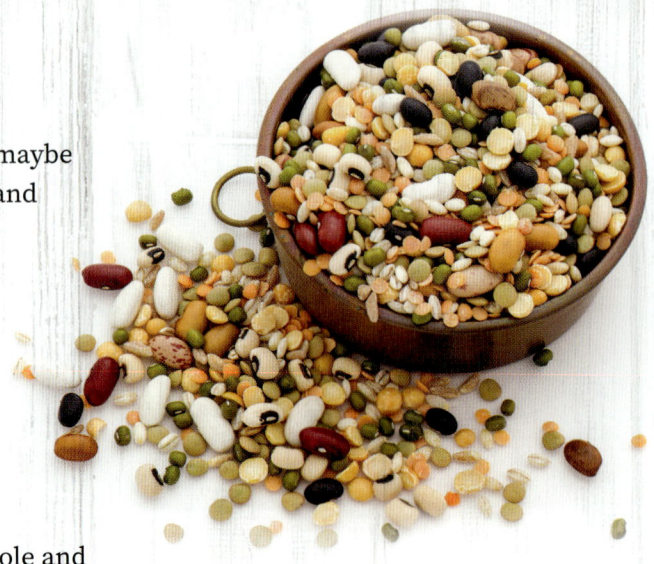

There are black beans, and red beans and white beans. But wait, maybe chick peas would be your favorite. And then there are split peas, and black-eyed peas, even peanuts are technically a legume. The variety of choices you have are many.

The nice part is the price. Beans are probably the healthiest foods on the planet and are literally the most cost effective. Dr. Michael Gregor has included them in his *Daily Dozen of Foods* that you should eat everyday.

The other thing I really like about beans and legumes is the fact that they can be served in different forms. You can keep them whole and firm, or mash them, even blend them into soups and sauces. What fun! With full on nutrition! It's a win win for the beans and legumes that you should be eating them every day.

BUTLER SOY CURLS

Butler Soy Curls would have to be my #1 choice for a vegan meat substitute. They are a dehydrated product that come with a lot of benefits. First of all, they are light weight, and when you rehydrate them, pound for pound it is less expensive than chicken.

On the nutrition side, they are made of non-GMO whole soy beans. That means you're getting all the good stuff. And they are filled with nutrients. With 11 grams of good protein, 6 grams of fiber, and only 5 grams of natural fat, this product should be a staple in your home too.

The product itself can be used in a wide range of applications. Your imagination will soar with everything from fajita meat, to soups and stews. We also love to just sauté them up crispy, to scatter on top of any salad.

To order a full case, visit this site and tell them Mark Anthony sent you.

https://www.butlerfoods.com || 503-437-9133

JACKFRUIT

Yes, it is actually a fruit, but you would never know it from the texture. This is a go to product when you are looking for that shredded look.

There are two different types of canned jackfruit. One is in a brine which is what I use for all of my meat substitute recipes. The other is packed in syrup, and used primarily for dessert recipes.

The nice part about jackfruit is that it has an extremely mild flavor that can be easily transformed into your own creations.

In addition to the 3 grams of protein per serving and the 40 grams of healthy carbs, jackfruit is loaded with vitamin C, and Magnesium. Even the calorie count is pretty good at 155 calories per cup.

LENTILS

Lentils are actually not a bean. Technically, Lentils are a grain legume known as a pulse because they are harvested for their seeds. Regardless of how you categorize them, they have played a vital roll in nutrition ever since the vegan movement began.

Loaded with healthy carbs, fiber and protein, the lentils will lead the way to an amazingly healthier you.

And they're not just for soup. Use the lentils for a meat substitute in tacos, and meatless loafs or lentil burgers. With a variety of colors and flavor, the price is right because a few lentils can go a long way. You simply can't go wrong with lentils.

MUSHROOMS

Mushrooms are a great way to get a meaty flavor and texture into your dishes. The Portobello mushrooms seem to get the customers award for flavor, but in all reality, it is simply a mature white button, or Cremini mushroom.

Another great mushroom is the King Oyster Mushroom. Available at most Asian food stores, the King Oyster is generally a lower price and has a much tougher meat - like stringy texture, and an amazing resemblance to fat when you eat it. I have used these for many meat substitute recipes.

Regardless of what mushrooms you use, they are sure to please, and they have a higher protein content that many people are searching for.

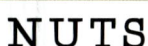

NUTS

Nuts are an excellent source of protein, therefore a common meat replacement.

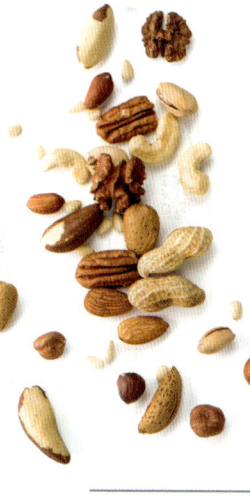

Chopped or ground, nuts can add texture and flavor to many dishes. Walnuts and Pecans have a reputation of great culinary value when it comes to meat substitutes in meat-less loaves, and casserole dishes.

Nuts provide the healthy fats and a combination of nutrients that are essential for healthy brain function. But be careful as they will also add many calories to the table.

SEITAN

Seitan has a very meaty texture. It is a gluten product, so people with celiac disease can't consume it. Seitan is also a great source of protein.

Depending on how you prepare it, Seitan can be similar to beef, chicken, or pork. You can make the texture chewy or soft. The texture can hold up to many cooking applications, even baking and frying. Plus it is really easy to create a variety of flavors.

TEMPEH

Tempeh can generally be found in most grocery stores, next to the tofu. It is firmer than tofu and has more texture, some being very grainy or marbled. Unlike the bland flavor of tofu, Tempeh has a nutty flavor. Made from fermented soy-beans, it's packed with protein as well as fiber, calcium, and vitamins.

Tempeh is easy to use, no pressing needed. Just slice it, chop it, or dice it. If you find Tempeh to be a little bitter, you can try steaming it for a few minutes before using.

It is a great substitute for ground beef. Use it in chili and other casserole dishes. Also simply slicing and pan frying it works great for sandwiches. Try it with BBQ sauce!

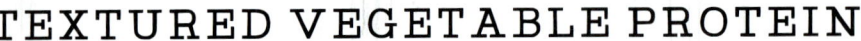

TEXTURED VEGETABLE PROTEIN

Textured vegetable protein is often known as TVP. It's a dehydrated soy product that is basically the remains of soybeans, after the oil is removed. Once you rehydrate it, you can use it for many applications.

One of the most popular ways to use it is simply as a burger substitute for tacos, or in chili. If you add a binder to it, you can make burgers and meatloaf. It doesn't have much flavor, so be sure to have the spices on hand to customize to your tastes.

TOFU

I would recommend having tofu as a staple in your refrigerator. Purchase the fresh, water packed as well as the more shelf stable silken version in a box. It's fast and easy to make a tofu egg salad, or bake off some tofu bacon. And not only can you use it for a meat substitute, it can also be blended for sauces, smoothies, and desserts.

Tofu is made from soybeans and is high in protein and calcium. It has been a staple of Asian cuisine for generations. Most people think of tofu when they hear the words vegetarian or vegan. And they automat-ically think of a dry, tasteless product. In all reality, tofu can take on many different flavors. As far as the texture goes, tofu can be turned into a liquid, or when baked become as tough as leather.

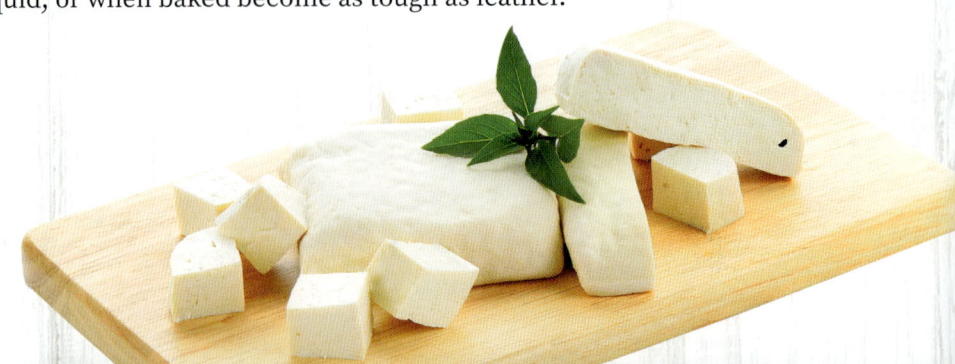

RECIPES

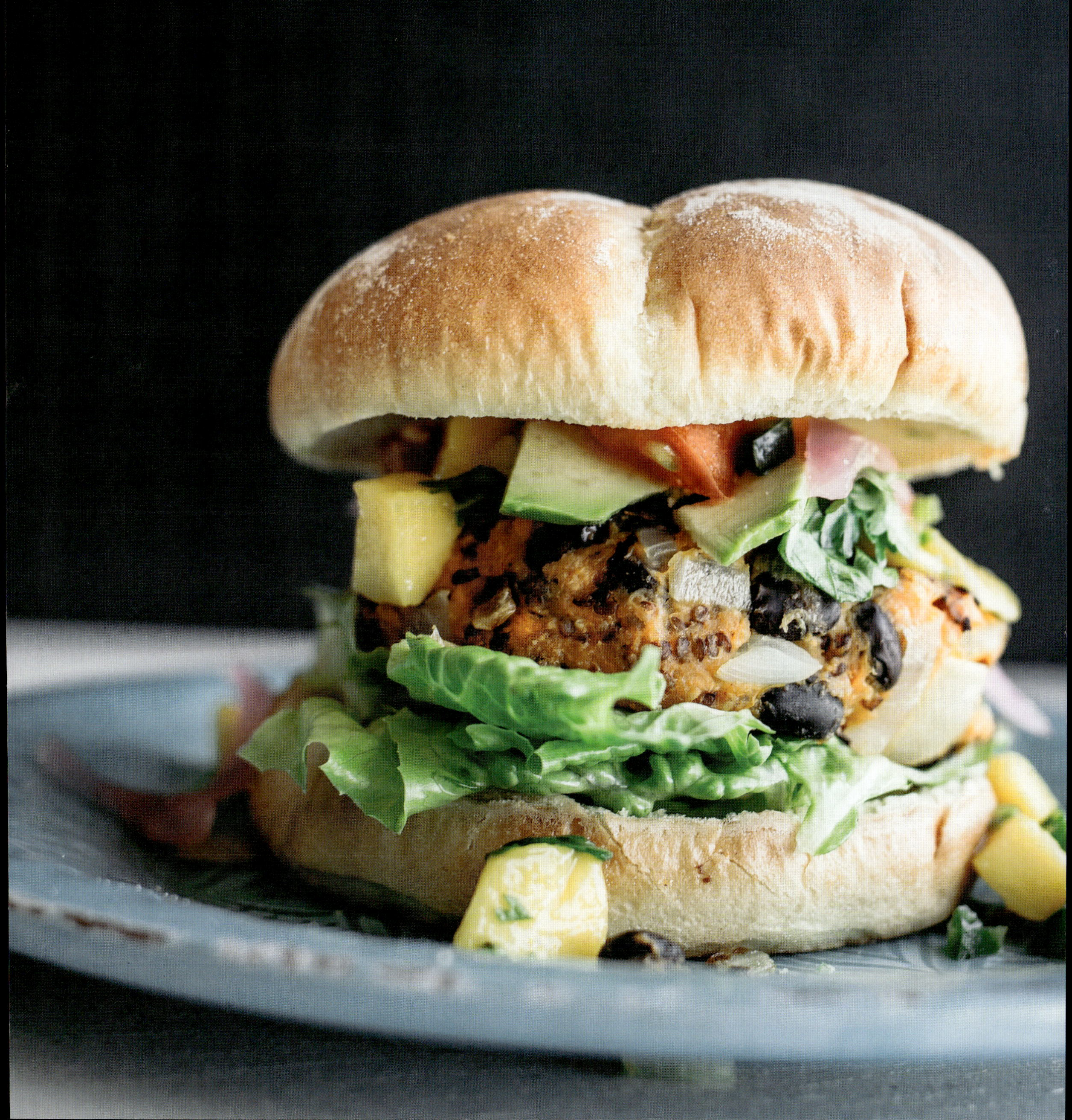

AFRICAN STEWED OXTAIL

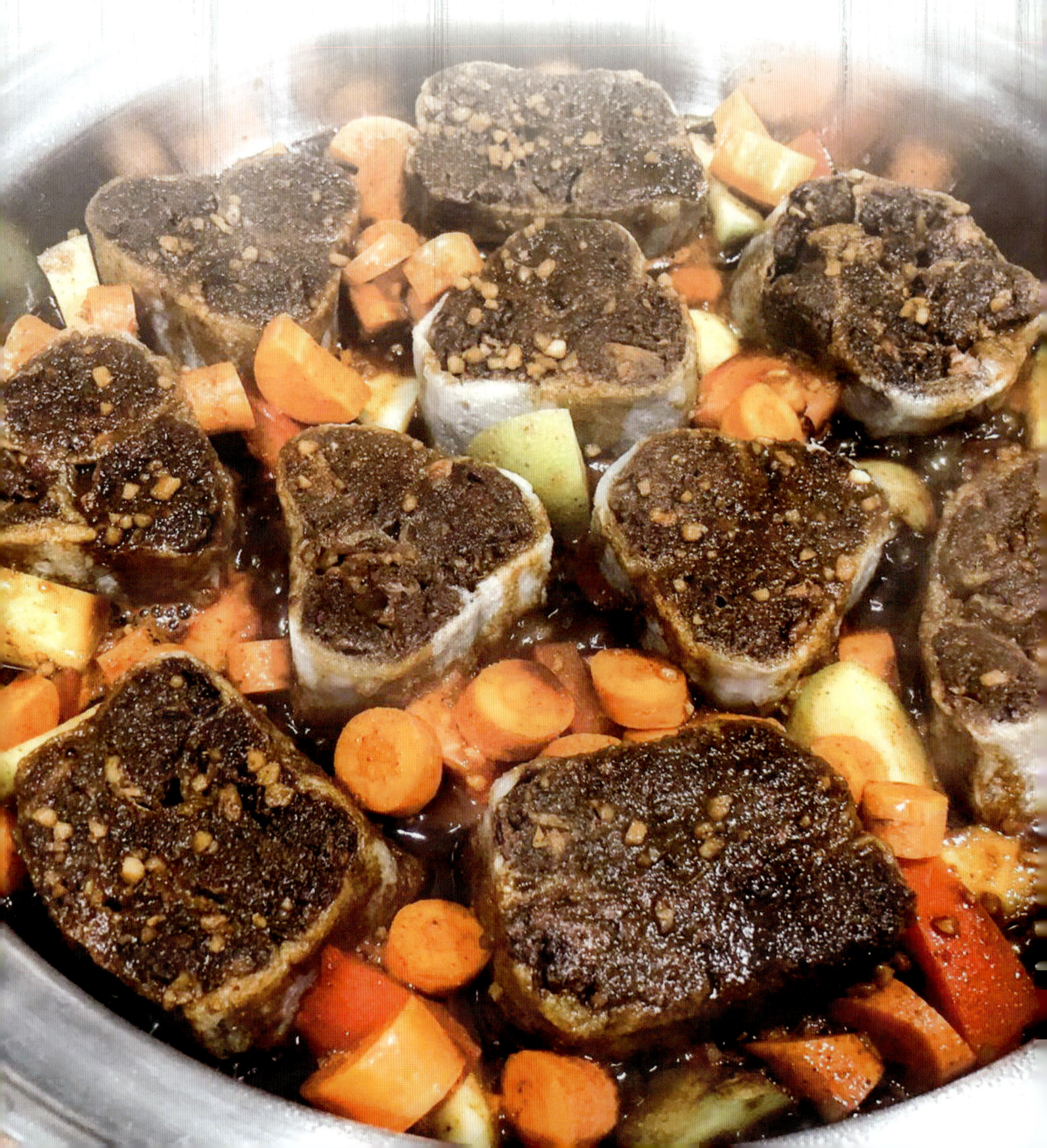

AFRICAN STEWED OXTAIL

On our trip to Africa, this was on the menu at one of the restaurants we visited. I determined to create a vegan version, and this is it. A near perfect clone of meat, without all the unhealthy side effects. Your guests will be absolutely amazed at how realistic this dish really is.

YIELD: 10 SERVINGS	PREP TIME: 25 MINUTES	COOKING TIME: 1.5 HOURS

ingredients

2 King Oyster mushrooms
1 can jack fruit

wet mix

1/2 cup water
2 Tbsp beef-less base
2 Tbsp soy sauce
2 Tbsp olive oil
1/2 Tbsp garlic
1 tsp onion powder
1 tsp chili powder
1/2 tsp salt
1/8 tsp caramel color

dry mix

1 1/2 c Vital wheat gluten
1/4 cup almond flour

additional ingredients

10 sheets rice paper, 9-inch square
vegetable broth mixture   *(see next page)*

directions

1. The first thing you are going to do is boil the king oyster mushrooms and jack fruit. I like to make sure they are covered with water. Bring to a boil and then simmer for 30 minutes.
2. When they are done, you can cool under cold running water.
3. Shred the mushrooms and the jack fruit into finely shredded one inch pieces.
4. Mix the wet ingredients with the shredded "meat".
5. Add the dry ingredients and mix well.
6. Divide into 6 equal parts.
7. Form into logs and wrap in one or two sheets of rice paper that has been softened with water. The "meat" needs to be equal thickness from one end of the rice paper log to the other end.
8. After you have the 6 logs, you are going to bundle 3 of them together and wrap again with 2 more sheets of rice paper. Keep it tight.
9. Sear the logs on all sides just enough to seal the rice paper. You can do this in your skillet with a little bit of oil in the pan.
10. Cut these 2 logs into 5 pieces each for a total of 10 oxtail steaks.
11. Place the oxtails in a skillet, cut side down.
12. Add the vegetables and broth mixture *(see next page)* and cook at 190° F for 1 hour. Flip the oxtails half way through the cooking process. Skillet temperatures vary. With the lid on the skillet, you want to have it at a very low simmer. And the volume of liquid should be about half way up the oxtails.
13. The oxtails are ready to serve.

Chef's Notes

These oxtail are great for freezing. I will generally wrap 3 at a time with saran wrap and then foil; and then write with a marker the item and date. This is a fun recipe that will really freak out anybody that is a little squeamish about eating meat. But they taste fantastic, so if you have to call them *Mushroom and Jack Fruit Pinwheels,* go ahead!

Watch the recipe here

VEGETABLE BROTH MIXTURE

This mixture pairs perfectly with the African Stewed Oxtail on the previous page.

ingredients

2 cups chopped carrots
2 cups chopped potatoes
1 cup diced tomatoes
1 cup chopped celery
1 cup water
2 Tbsp ketchup
2 Tbsp soy sauce
1 Tbsp beef-less base
1 Tbsp Kitchen bouquet
1 Tbsp molasses
1 Tbsp minced garlic
1 tsp chili powder
1 tsp cumin
1 tsp smoked paprika
1 tsp onion powder
1 tsp ginger
1 tsp turmeric
1 tsp salt
1/4 tsp liquid smoke
2 jalapeños sliced (optional)

directions

1. Chop up the vegetables, and mix all ingredients together.
2. See the previous page for the finishing instructions.

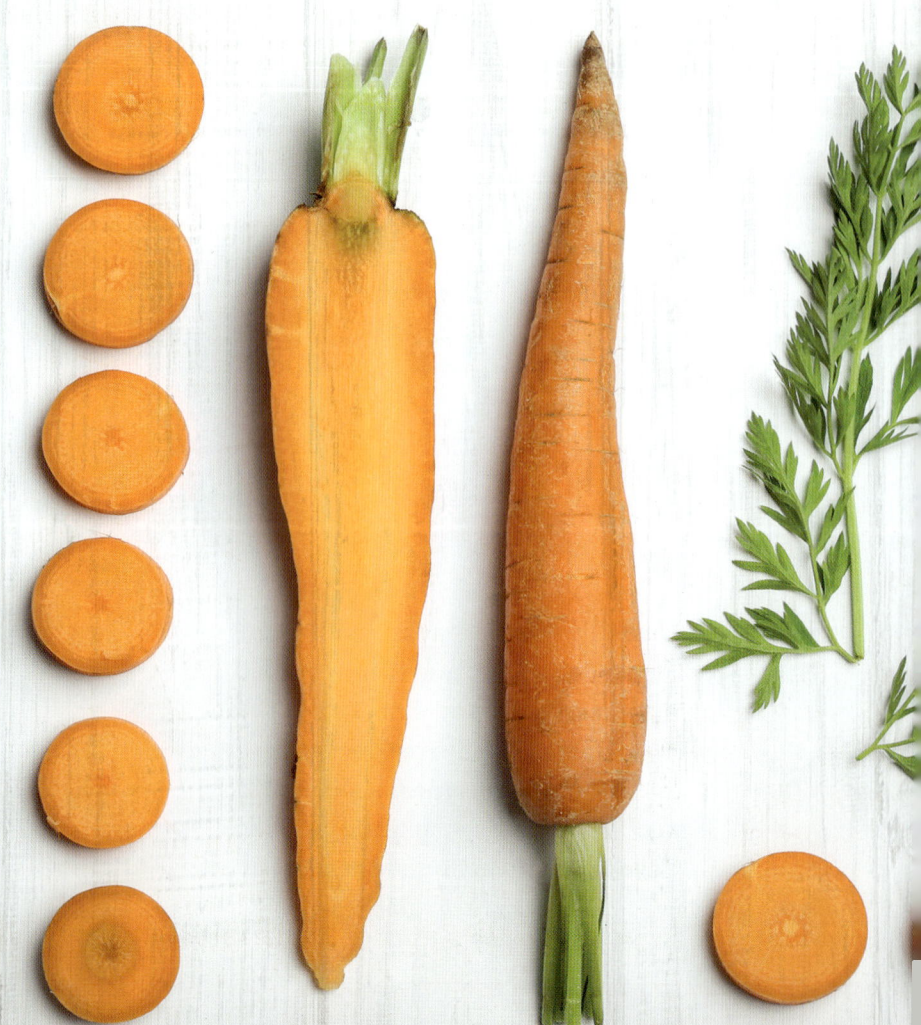

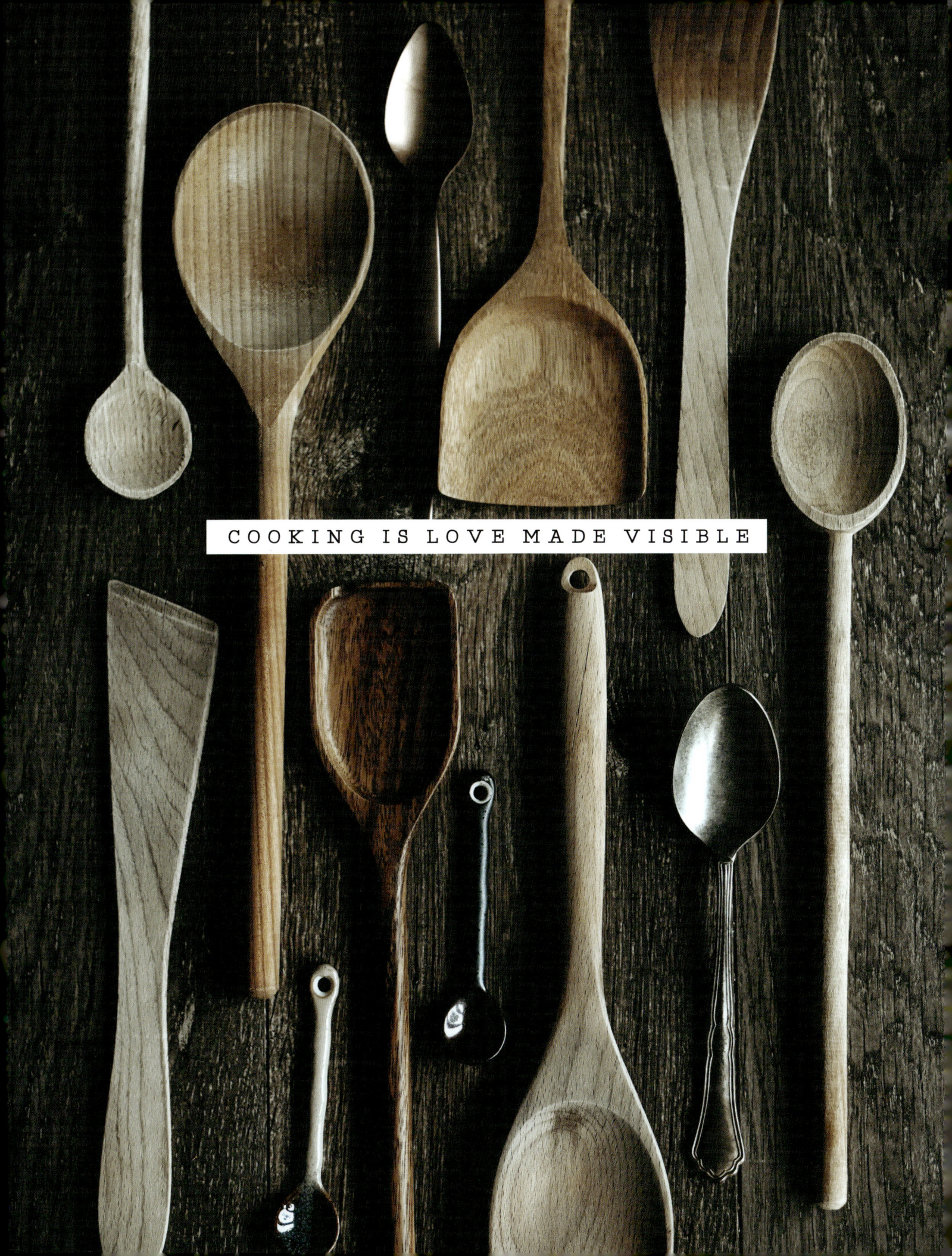

COOKING IS LOVE MADE VISIBLE

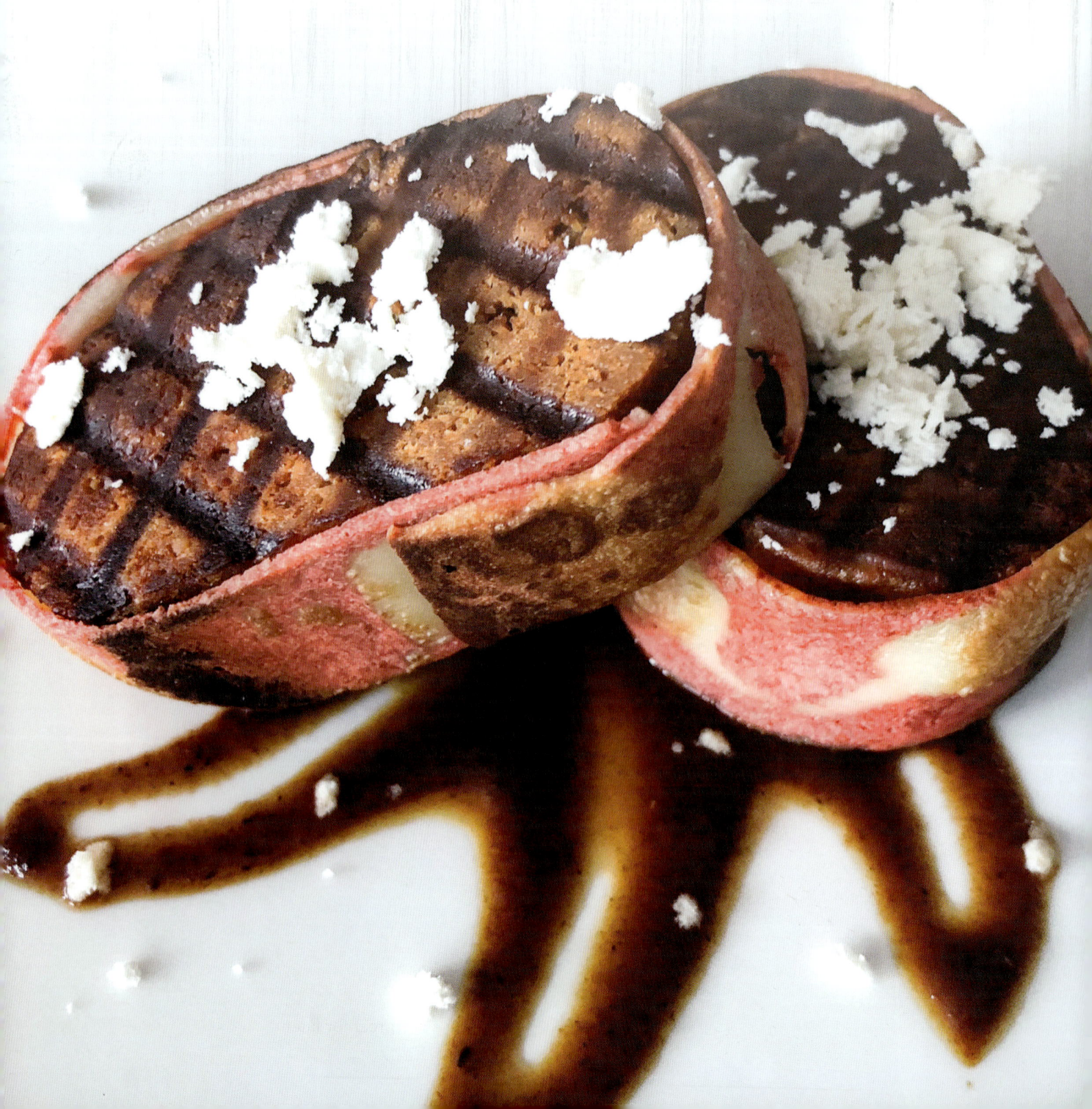

BACON WRAPPED FILET MIGNON

The flavor of this creation definitely makes it one of my five star recipes.

YIELD: 16 SERVINGS	PREP TIME: 20 MINUTES	COOKING TIME: 1 HOUR

wet ingredients

3 cups chick peas (2 -15oz cans, rinsed and drained)
2 cups water
1 1/2 cups tomato paste
1/2 cup soy sauce
1/2 cup nutritional yeast flakes
1/2 cup smoked paprika
1/4 cup olive oil
2 Tbsp fresh, chopped garlic
2 Tbsp A-1 steak sauce
2 Tbsp brown mustard
2 Tbsp beef-less base
2 Tbsp onion powder
2 Tbsp garlic powder
1 Tbsp beet powder (optional)

dry ingredients

5 cups Vital wheat gluten four
1 cup rice flour
2 Tbsp xanthan gum

additional ingredients

steak seasoning
Vegan bacon strips

directions

1. Pre-heat oven to 350°F.
2. Blend the wet ingredients in a food processor until almost smooth. A little lumpy is okay.
3. In an extra large bowl, mix the dry ingredients.
4. Combine the wet with the dry. Mix together very well.
5. Divide into 2 portions. And roll them into logs that would have the diameter of a filet mignon.
6. Place the logs into a parchment lined hotel pan or extra large casserole dish.
7. Cover with steak seasoning then add about 2 cups of water into the pan and cover with foil.
8. Bake for 45 minutes covered, and then another 15 minutes uncovered.
9. Allow to rest before cutting.
10. From here, you can charbroil, or I use a panini grill to give them some nice markings.
11. Wrap steaks with vegan bacon. You will want to pan fry the bacon wrapped steaks on their sides to brown the bacon.

Watch the recipe here

Chef's Notes

I recommend watching the video on this one so you can really grasp the concept. This is a bigger volume recipe, because it is great for later use and freezing.

BARON OF BEEF

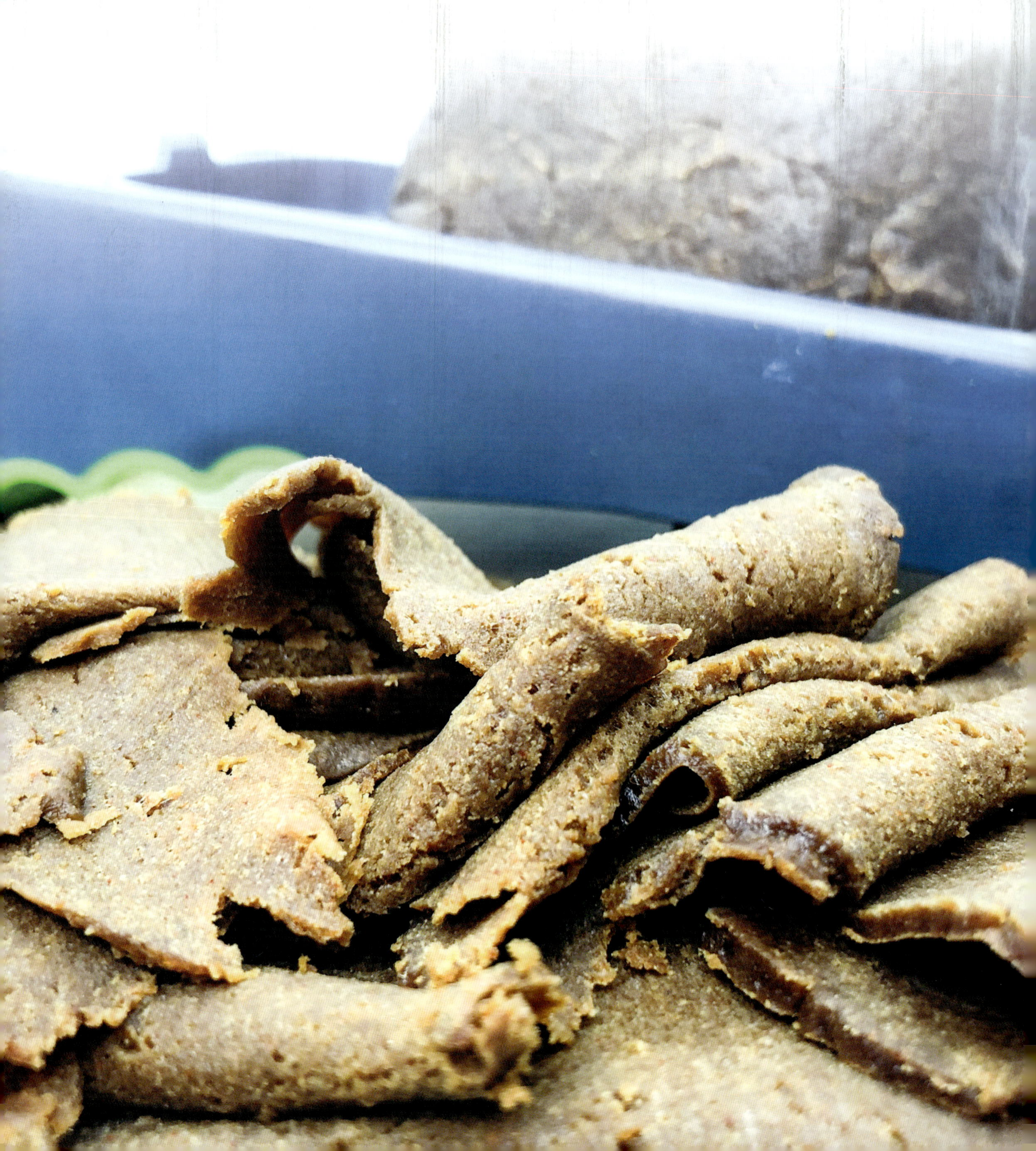

BARON OF BEEF

This recipe really captures the texture of beef, with a fraction of the fat. You can slice it thick or thin.

YIELD: 12 SERVINGS	PREP TIME: 20 MINUTES	COOKING TIME: 1.5 HOURS

wet ingredients

1/2 cup water
1/2 cup soy sauce
1/4 cup A-1 steak sauce
2 Tbsp olive oil
2 Tbsp beef-less base
2 Tbsp onion powder
1 Tbsp garlic powder
1 Tbsp browning liquid (Kitchen Bouquet)
1 Tbsp liquid smoke
1 Tbsp brown sugar
drop caramel color (optional)

dry ingredients

2 cups Vital wheat gluten flour
1/4 cup millet flour
1 Tbsp smoked paprika
2 Tbsp tapioca starch
2 Tbsp xanthan gum

directions

1. Preheat oven to 350°F.
2. Blend the wet ingredients.
3. In a large bowl, mix the dry ingredients.
4. Combine the wet and dry ingredients and mix well.
5. Wrap tight with parchment paper and then foil wrap 2 times, forming into a flatter shape rather than round.
6. Place in a casserole dish with about 1/2 inch of water in the bottom.
7. I also place another casserole pan on top of the beef to help hold the shape.
8. Bake for 1 1/2 hours.
9. Chill in foil over night and it's ready to slice.

Watch the recipe here

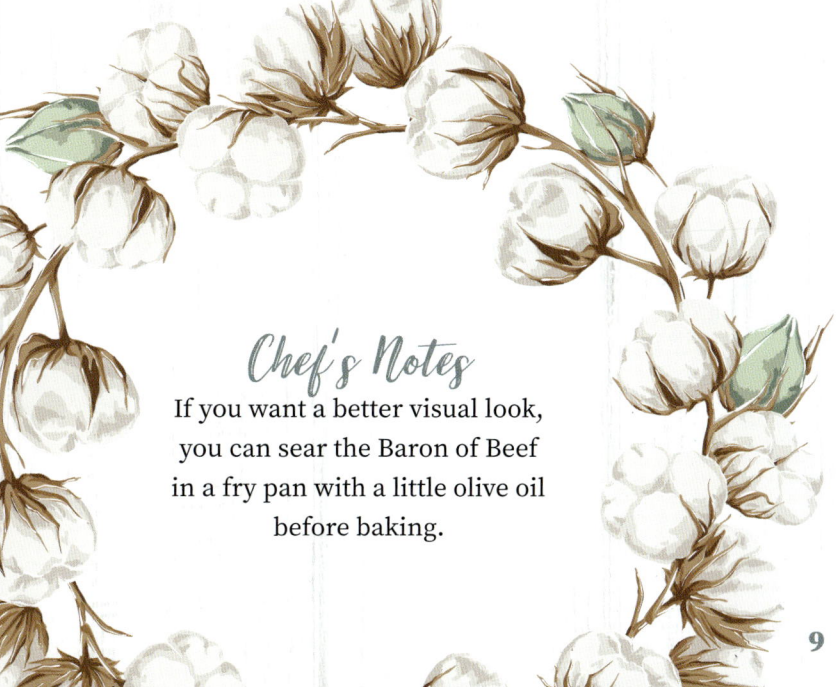

Chef's Notes

If you want a better visual look, you can sear the Baron of Beef in a fry pan with a little olive oil before baking.

BBQ CHICKEN FILET

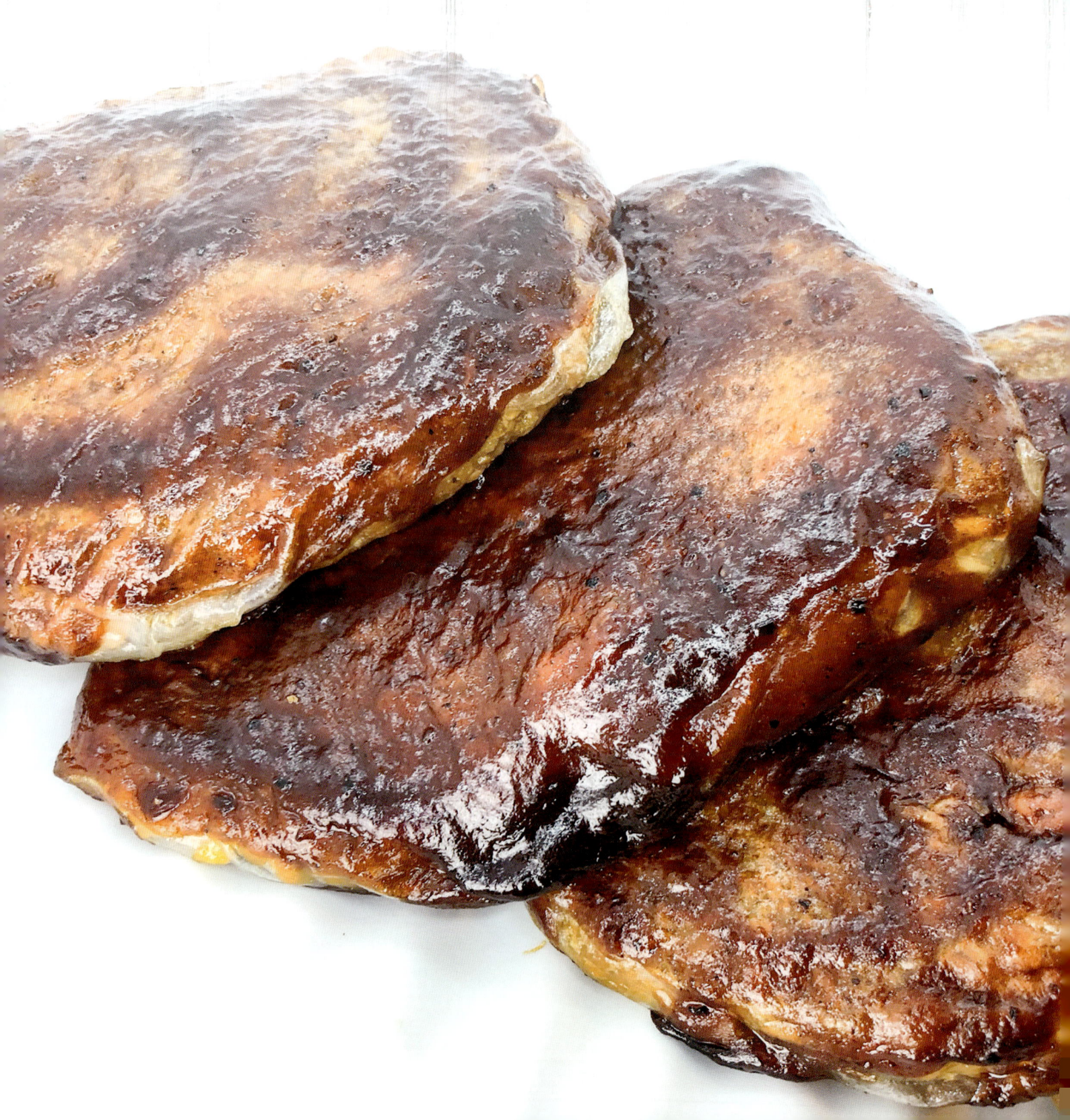

BBQ CHICKEN FILET

I've tried quite a few variables to create a perfect chicken style recipe with well over 3 dozen experiments. This is one of my favorites. It is relatively easy with great flavor and texture.

YIELD: 6 TO 8 SERVINGS	PREP TIME: 20 MINUTES	COOKING TIME: 1.5 HOURS

wet ingredients

1 can jack fruit
1 1/2 cups chick peas, cooked and drained
1/2 cup water
3 Tbsp olive oil
1/4 cup BBQ sauce
1 Tbsp soy sauce
1 Tbsp chicken-less base
1 Tbsp onion powder
1/2 Tbsp garlic powder
1 tsp poultry seasoning
2 tsp sugar
1 tsp salt

dry ingredients

1 1/2 cups Vital wheat gluten flour
1/4 cup nutritional yeast flakes
3 Tbsp rice flour

additional ingredients

6 sheets rice paper
1/2 cup BBQ sauce

Chef's Note

This recipe can be done without any BBQ sauce. And you can jazz up the flavors by using teriyaki, or simply making a chicken style dry rub to coat them with.

directions

1. Boil off the jack fruit in water for 30 minutes, then run cold water over it to chill.
2. Preheat the oven to 350°F.
3. Squeeze all the moisture you can out of the jack fruit and then shred it.
4. In a large bowl, smash the chickpeas with a fork
5. Add the remaining wet ingredients with the jack fruit and chick peas, and mix well
6. In another bowl, mix the dry together.
7. Combine the wet and the dry ingredients, and mix well. You will want to mix this for a good 2-3 minutes. This will get the gluten to have some elasticity.
8. Divide into 6 or 7 pieces and shape like a chicken breast with one side thicker than the other.
9. Place the rice paper on a wet cutting board to soften, one sheet at a time. Then wrap the chicken breasts with the rice paper, making sure the rice paper comes together to enclose the chicken.
10. Pan fry the chicken breasts on each side to seal the rice paper together.
11. Place on a parchment lined sheet pan, and splash with your favorite BBQ sauce.
12. Bake for a total of 40 minutes. Every 10 minutes you will want to flip and baste with a little more BBQ sauce.
13. These are ready to serve or may be chilled and saved for later use.

Watch the recipe here

BBQ CHICKEN SANDWICH

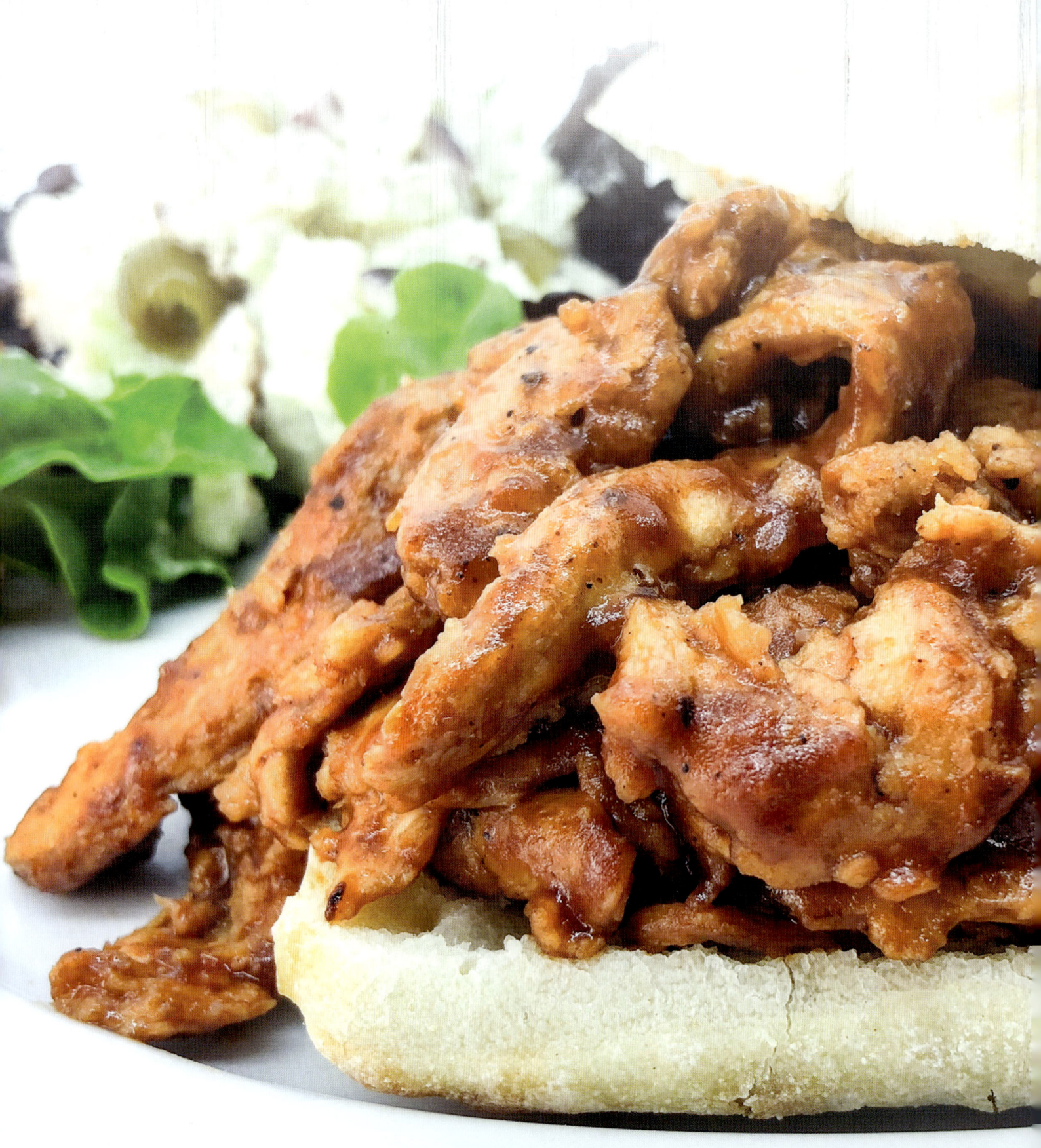

BBQ CHICKEN SANDWICH

GLUTEN FREE WITH BUTLER SOY CURLS

This is an easy recipe that you are going to want to keep in your regular menu rotation.
I've taken BBQ flavor to a whole new dimension with the Asian flair of ginger and fresh garlic.

| YIELD: 6 SERVINGS | PREP TIME: 10 MINUTES | COOKING TIME: 40 MINUTES |

EAST MEETS WEST BBQ SAUCE

ingredients

1 cup ketchup
1 cup water
1 onion, finely chopped (about 1/2 cup)
1/2 cup red wine vinegar
1/4 cup brown sugar
2 garlic cloves, minced
2 tsp fresh grated ginger
1/4 tsp salt

additional ingredients

2 cups butler soy curls, rehydrated and drained
Your favorite gluten-free bun or bread

directions

1. In a medium sauce pan, combine all the BBQ sauce ingredients over a medium heat. Stir constantly for 5 minutes. Reduce heat to low and simmer for 20 minutes, stirring occasionally. The sauce should be good and thick.
2. Add the rehydrated soy curls, and simmer for another 10 minutes.
3. It's ready to serve or chill for later use.

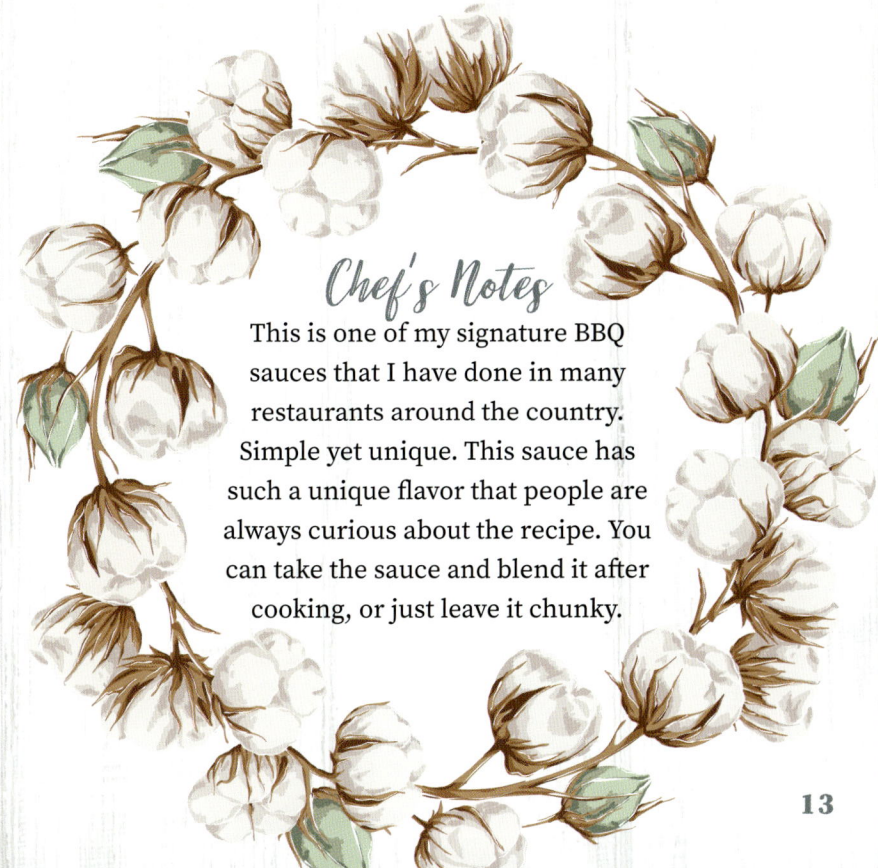

Chef's Notes

This is one of my signature BBQ sauces that I have done in many restaurants around the country. Simple yet unique. This sauce has such a unique flavor that people are always curious about the recipe. You can take the sauce and blend it after cooking, or just leave it chunky.

Watch the recipe here

BBQ PORK SANDWICHES

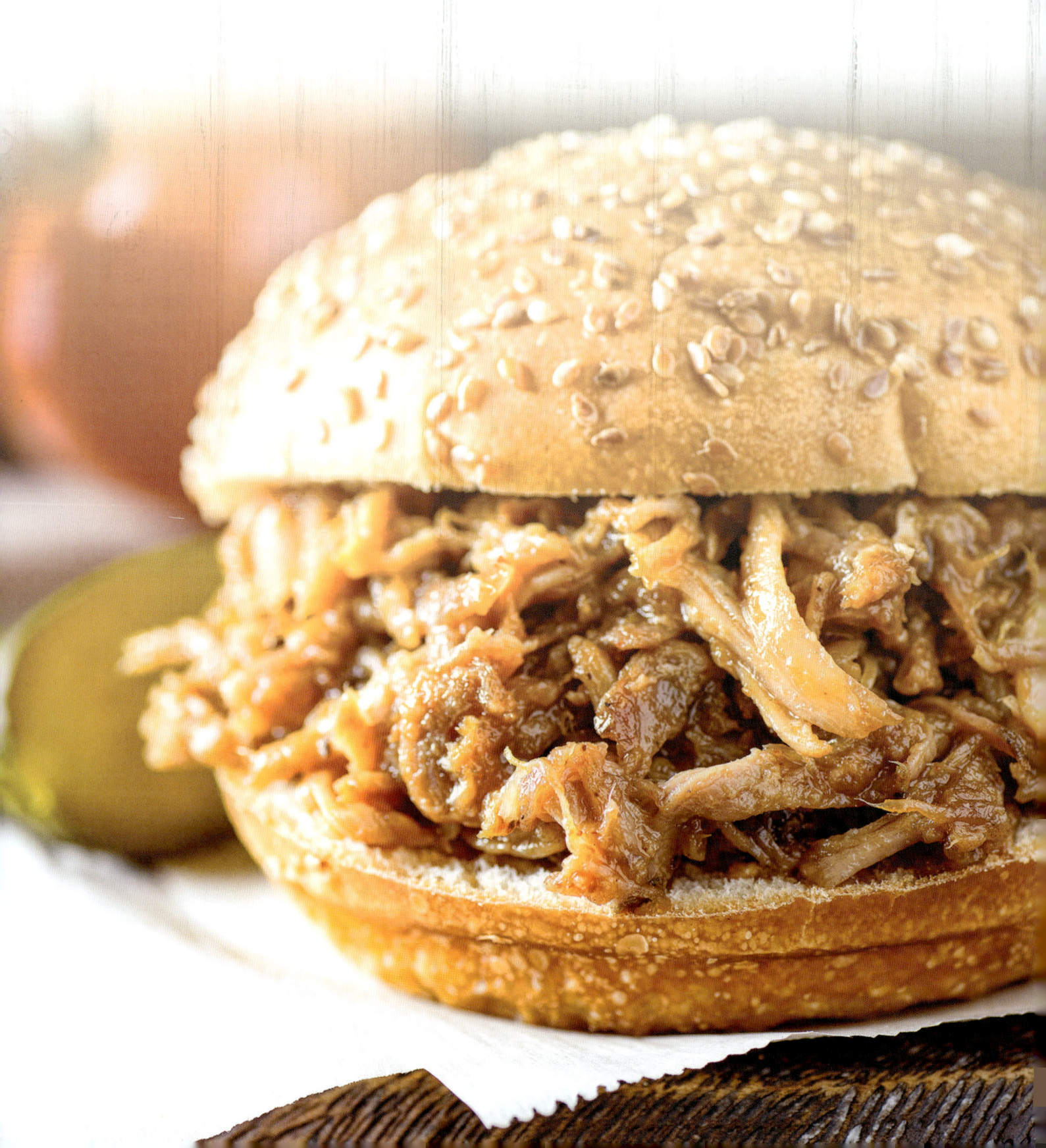

BBQ PORK SANDWICHES

This is my simplest vegan meat recipe of all. And it is so good, you will put this on your regular menu.

YIELD: 4 TO 6 SERVINGS	PREP TIME: 10 MINUTES	COOKING TIME: 40 MINUTES

ingredients

2 cans jack fruit in brine
BBQ Sauce

directions

1. Boil off the jack fruit for 30 minuses
2. Drain and then mash up the fruit. You can do this by hand or with a knife.
3. Add BBQ sauce and cook on medium heat until it reduces to desired thickness.

HONEY JERK BBQ SAUCE

This BBQ sauce is the perfect combination of BBQ and Caribbean.

ingredients

1 cup honey
3 oz tomato paste
1/4 cup brown sugar
1 Tbsp jerk seasoning
1/2 Tbsp dijon mustard
1/2 Tbsp garlic powder
 dash Tabasco

directions

Combine all ingredients, bring to a boil. Remove from heat and let rest till completely cool.

Watch the recipe here

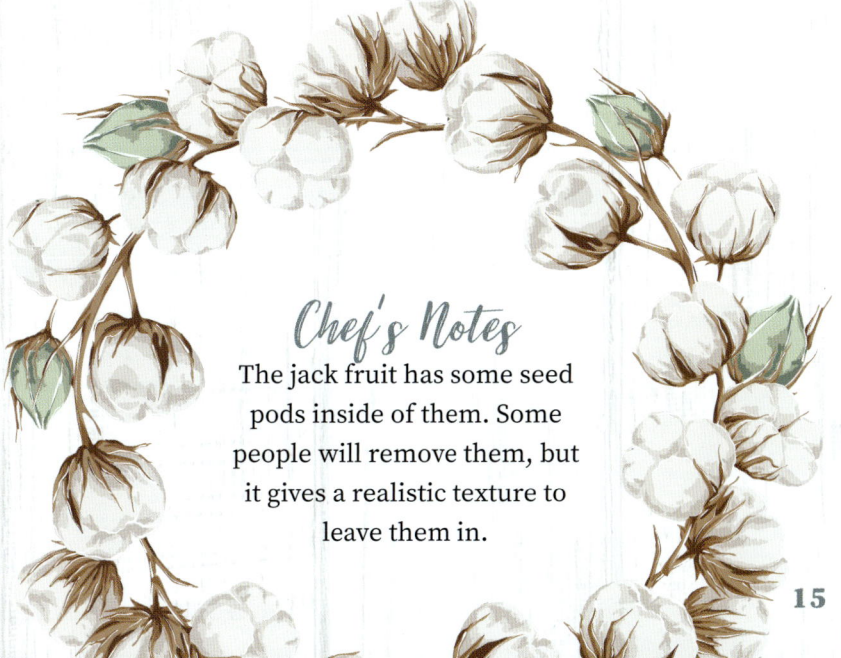

Chef's Notes

The jack fruit has some seed pods inside of them. Some people will remove them, but it gives a realistic texture to leave them in.

BBQ SHORT RIBS - BONELESS

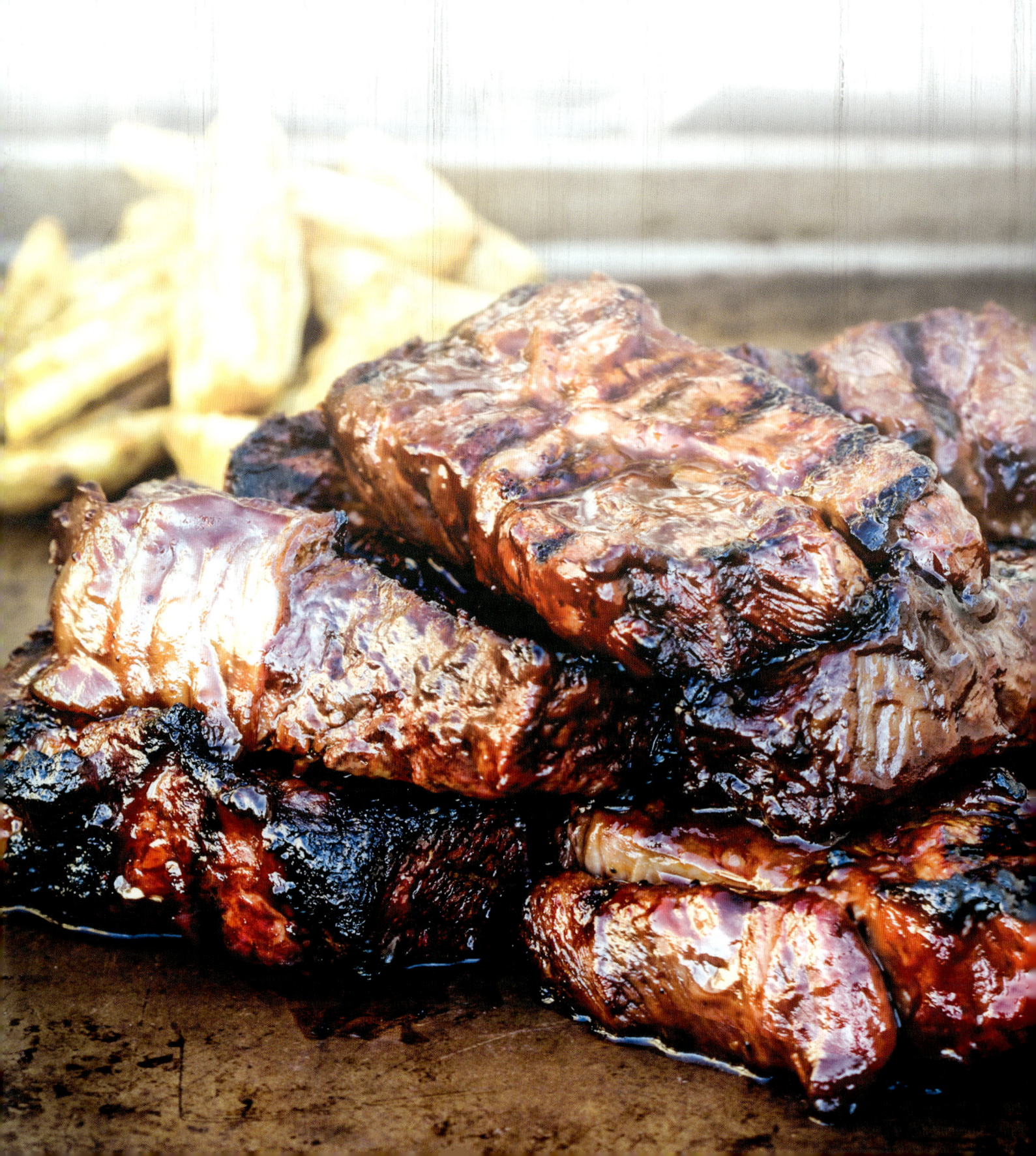

BBQ SHORT RIBS
BONELESS

This recipe is definitely a winner! The texture is just like short ribs, the flavor is just like short ribs, and the look is just like short ribs. It took many attempts to perfect this recipe.
There are a few steps, but most of the time is in the cooking and not the prep.

YIELD: 6 SERVINGS	PREP TIME: 20 MINUTES	COOKING TIME: 2 HOURS

ingredients

3 King oyster mushrooms
1 can jackfruit in brine

bbq rub

1/2 cup ketchup
1/4 cup water
1/4 cup olive oil
1/2 cup brown sugar
2 Tbsp spicy brown mustard
1 Tbsp hickory liquid smoke
1 Tbsp smoked paprika
1 Tbsp chili powder
1 Tbsp onion powder
1 tsp garlic powder
1 tsp cumin
1 tsp sea salt
1/4 tsp cayenne

SEITAN MIXTURE
wet mixture

1 1/2 cups water
2 Tbsp Kitchen Bouquet
3 Tbsp Better than Bouillon Beef-less base
1/4 cup "BBQ Rub" (the rub used on the mushrooms)
1/4 tsp carmel color (optional)

dry mixture

2 1/2 cups Vital wheat gluten flour
1/2 cup chickpea flour

additional ingredients

6 rice paper sheets 9-inch

Watch the recipe here

directions

1. Mix all the ingredients for the BBQ rub together.
2. Take the 6 king oyster mushrooms and cut in half length-wise. Rub generously with BBQ Rub. Place in baking dish and bake covered at 350°F for 1 hour. Remove and allow to cool.
3. Boil off the can of jackfruit for 30 minutes, then cool and shred into pieces.
4. Shred the mushrooms with a fork. These should be long stringy and very thin. Add this to the shredded jackfruit and mix well.
5. Next, make the seitan mixture by blending the liquid and adding it to the dry mixture.
6. Add the shredded mushrooms, jackfruit and mix well.
7. Divide into 6 equal portions.
8. Wrap each portion with a sheet of rice paper, softened with water.
9. Carefully rub with remaining BBQ rub. Bake for 45 minutes, flipping over 1/2 way through baking.
10. They are then ready to serve with your favorite BBQ sauce. Great to freeze or chill and reheat.

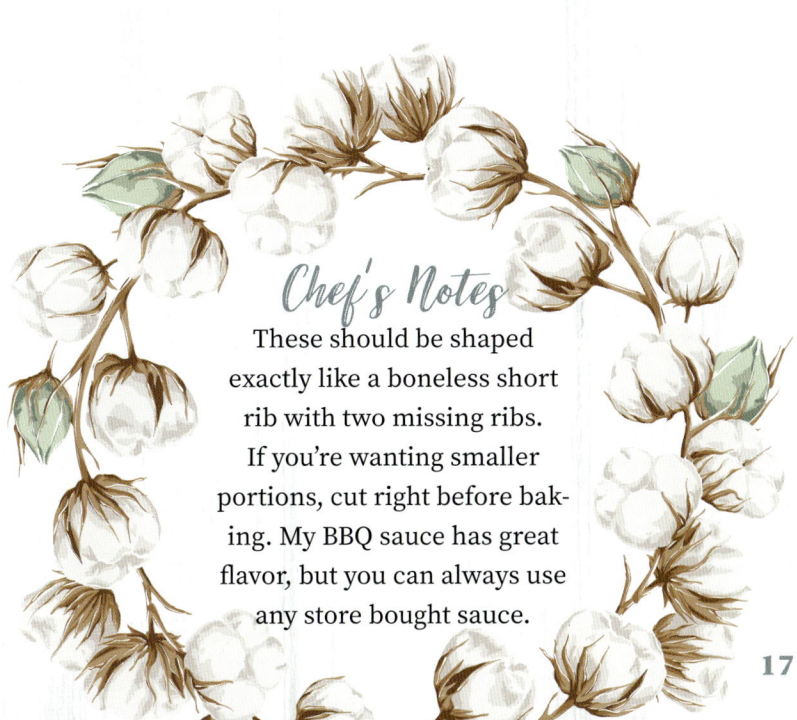

Chef's Notes

These should be shaped exactly like a boneless short rib with two missing ribs. If you're wanting smaller portions, cut right before baking. My BBQ sauce has great flavor, but you can always use any store bought sauce.

BEEF BRISKET GLUTEN FREE

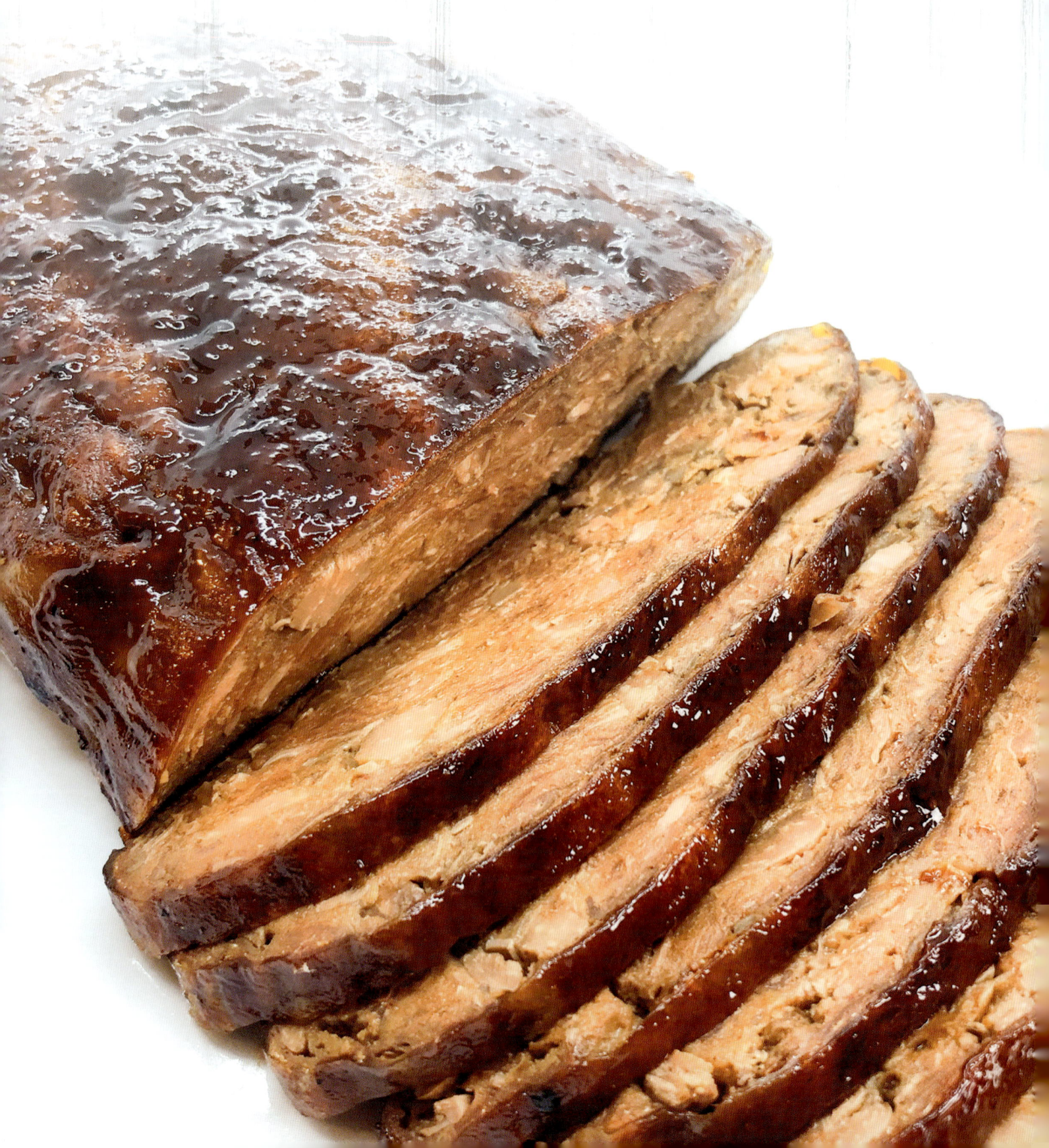

BEEF BRISKET
GLUTEN FREE

We have perfected this recipe to become one of the best vegan meat recipes you will ever enjoy.
And it's GLUTEN FREE. I've tried it with gluten flours, but this just worked better.

YIELD: 8 SERVINGS	PREP TIME: 25 MINUTES	COOKING TIME: 1.75 HOURS

wet ingredients

3 cans jackfruit, drained
4 cups water
1/4 cup tomato paste
1/4 soy sauce
1/4 cup brown sugar
1 Tbsp beef-less base
1 Tbsp liquid smoke
2 Tbsp smoked paprika
1 Tbsp chili powder
1 Tbsp onion powder
1 Tbsp garlic powder
1 Tbsp salt

dry ingredients

1 cup chickpea flour
1/4 cup rice flour
1/4 cup tapioca flour
2 Tbsp xanthan gum
2 Tbsp beet powder
5 sheets large rice paper, chopped

additional ingredients

4 sheets rice paper, 9-inch large
oil for frying

directions

1. Simmer the wet ingredients for 30 minutes.
2. Allow to cool in the juice.
3. Drain the jackfruit, reserving only 3/4 cup of the juice that it was cooked in.
4. Mash the jack fruit into a shredded consistency.
5. Chop or blend the rice paper sheets into small pieces, not powder. I have used both a food processor, and a coffee grinder. You will want to break them up a little bit first.
6. Mix the rice paper in with all the dry ingredients.
7. Mix together the dry ingredients with the jack fruit and reserved liquid.
8. Form into the shape of a brisket.
9. Wrap with the 4 rice paper sheets. You will want watch the video on this part. The rice paper needs to be wet in order to make it stretch. On a cutting board, taking two at a time and slightly overlapped, you will place the meat on top and then wrap, connecting the rice paper. Repeat the process on the other side.
10. Pan fry the brisket in a hot oiled pan. This will seal the rice paper.
11. On a parchment lined sheet pan, you will want to bake this at 350° F for about 75 minutes.
12. Splash some BBQ sauce on it, and flip and repeat half way through the cooking process.
13. Allow to cool, or refrigerate overnight, then slice. Reheat when ready to serve.

Chef's Notes

I like the 'Sticky Fingers' BBQ sauce. It is not made with high fructose corn syrup, and they have a couple different flavors. If you don't have the xanthan gum, double up on the tapioca flour.

Watch the recipe here

BRATWURST

BRATWURST

Traditional Bratwurst is made with pork and veal. None of that in this dish! This recipe is made with simple ingredients and is healthy and easy to produce.

YIELD: 4 TO 6 SERVINGS	PREP TIME: 15 MINUTES	COOKING TIME: 45 MINUTES

dry ingredients

1 cup Vital wheat gluten flour
1 Tbsp garbanzo bean flour
2 Tbsp tapioca starch
2 Tbsp onion powder
2 Tbsp chives, dried
1 Tbsp dried minced onions

wet ingredients

1 cup water
1/4 cup miso paste
2 Tbsp olive oil
2 Tbsp minced garlic
1 Tbsp sugar
1 tsp poultry seasoning
1 tsp ground caraway
1/2 tsp allspice
1/2 tsp nutmeg
1/2 tsp ginger
1 tsp salt

directions

1. Mix wet ingredients together.
2. Mix dry ingredients together in a separate bowl.
3. Combine the wet with the dry, and mix well.
4. Divide into 4 portions.
5. Tootsie roll wrap in both parchment paper and foil.
6. Steam for 45 min.
7. Cool in fridge overnight then unwrap reheat, or slice.

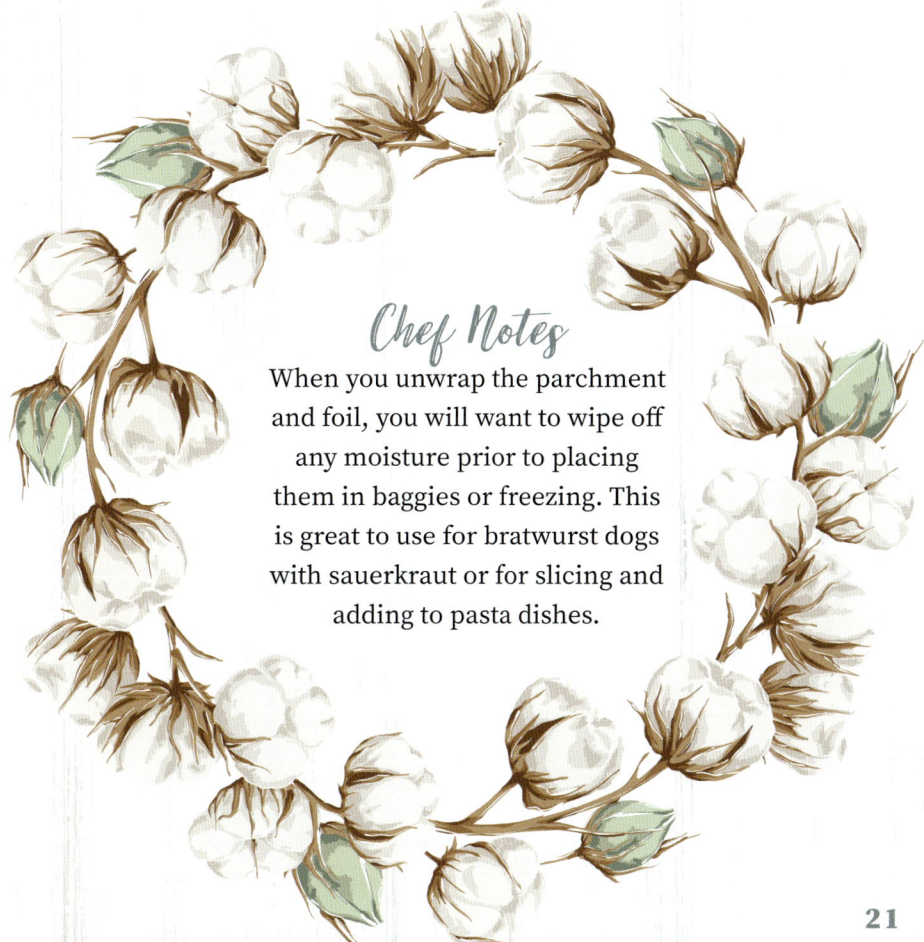

Chef Notes

When you unwrap the parchment and foil, you will want to wipe off any moisture prior to placing them in baggies or freezing. This is great to use for bratwurst dogs with sauerkraut or for slicing and adding to pasta dishes.

Watch the recipe here

BREADED CHICKEN NUGGETS

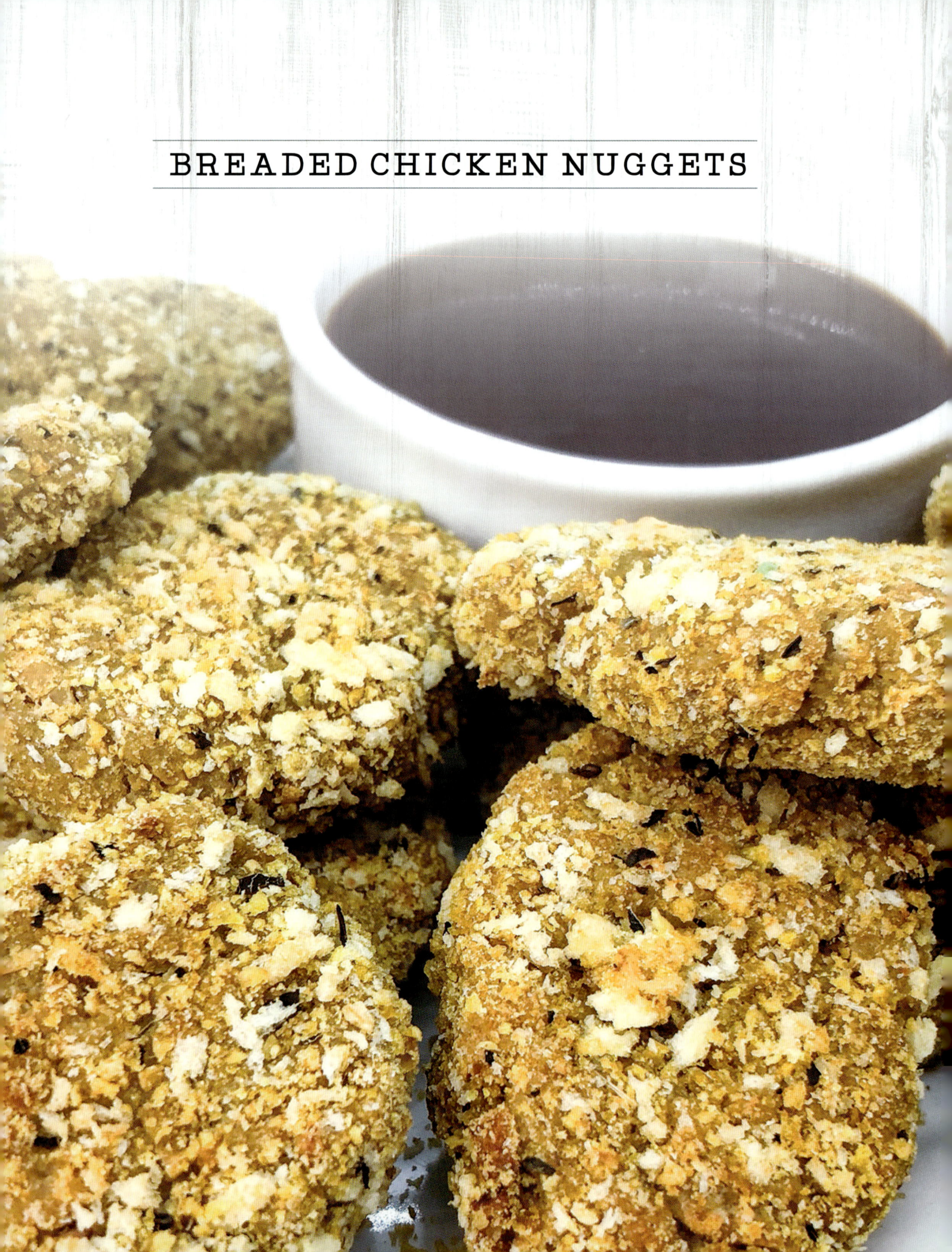

BREADED CHICKEN NUGGETS

This is simply a spin on my Breaded Chicken Sandwich recipe. Works perfect for chicken nuggets.

| YIELD: 16 TO 20 NUGGETS | PREP TIME: 20 MINUTES | COOKING TIME: 25 MINUTES |

wet ingredients

1 1/2 cups cooked and drained chick peas
1/2 cup water
2 Tbsp olive oil
2 Tbsp apple juice
1 Tbsp soy sauce
1 Tbsp apple cider vinegar
2 tsp chicken-less base
1 tsp onion powder
1/2 tsp garlic powder
1/2 tsp poultry seasoning
1 tsp sugar
1/2 tsp salt

dry ingredients

1 cup Vital wheat gluten flour
1/4 cup nutritional yeast flakes
2 Tbsp rice flour

breading ingredients

1/2 cup bread crumbs
1/2 cup Panko
1/2 Tbsp basil

directions

1. Preheat the oven to 400°F.
2. In a large bowl, smash the chickpeas with a fork
3. Add the remaining wet ingredients, and mix well
4. In another bowl, mix the dry ingredients together.
5. Combine the wet and the dry ingredients, and mix well. You will want to mix this for a good 2 minutes. This will get the gluten to have some elasticity.
6. Using a #30 scooper, we are going to form the portions into nugget size shapes. This will be a softer texture, but try to keep it tight.
7. Bread the nuggets by lightly pressing into the breading mixture.
8. Place on a parchment lined sheet pan, and mist with a little olive oil spray.
9. Bake for a total of 24 minutes. 12 minutes on one side, then flip, lightly spray again, then bake for another 12 minutes.
10. Best to cool on a wire rack, and serve while warm.

Watch the recipe here

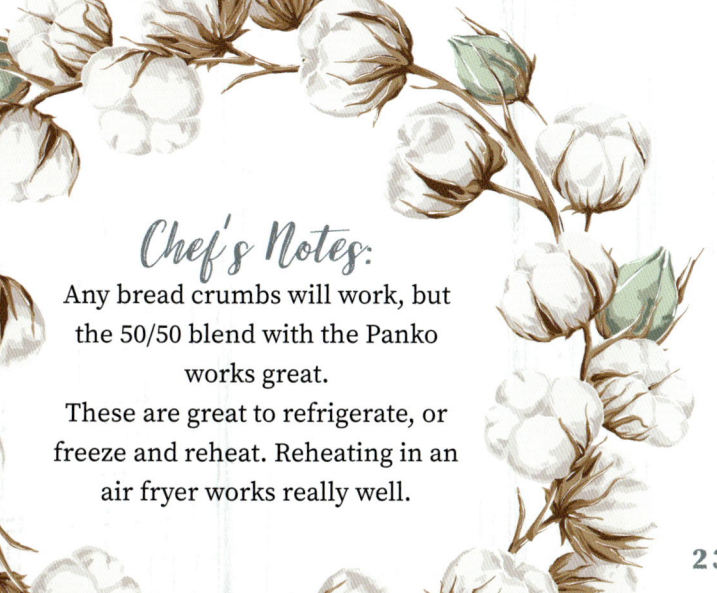

Chef's Notes:

Any bread crumbs will work, but the 50/50 blend with the Panko works great.
These are great to refrigerate, or freeze and reheat. Reheating in an air fryer works really well.

BREADED CHICKEN SANDWICH

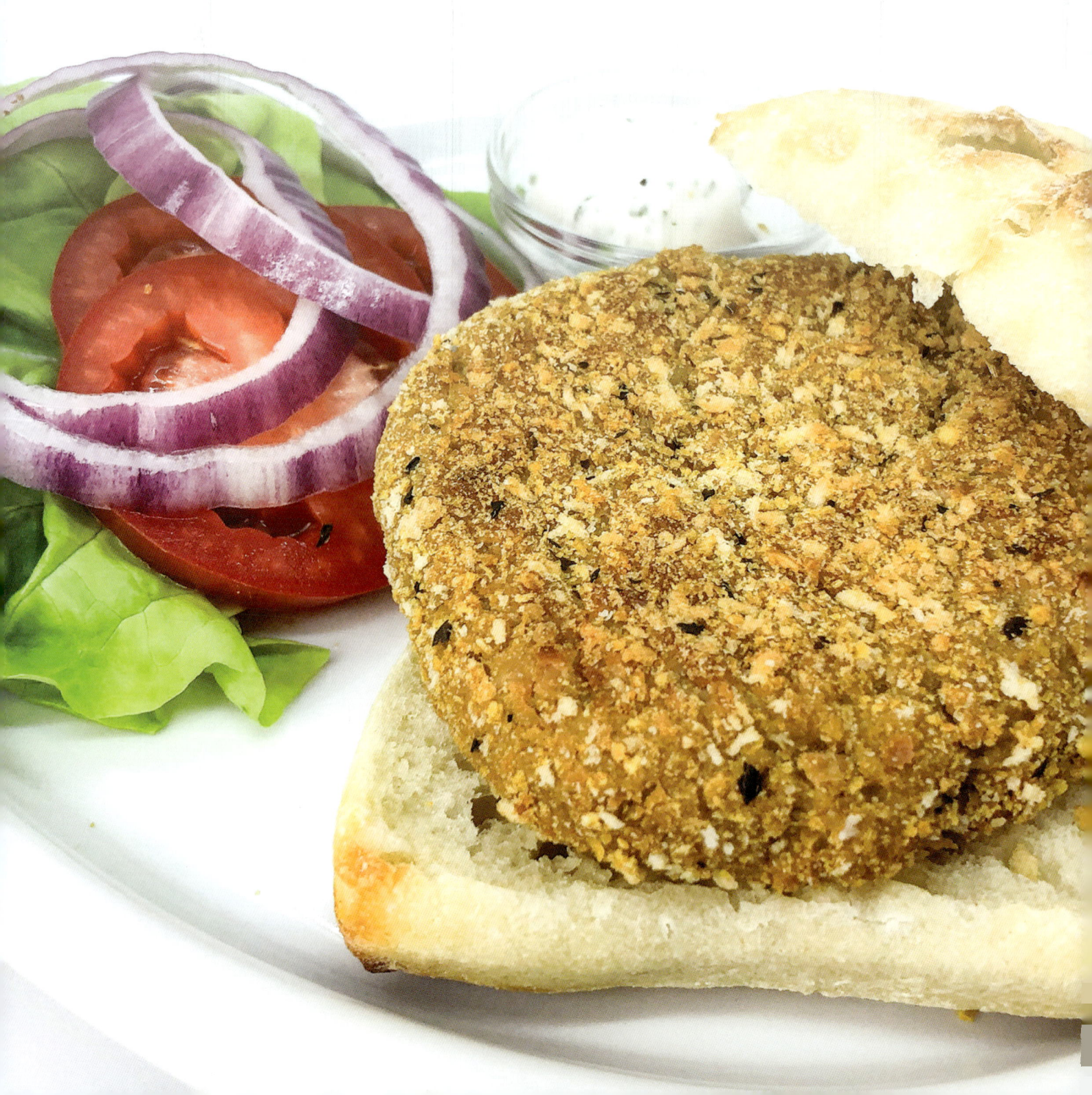

BREADED CHICKEN SANDWICH

This recipe is a home run. Yes it has great flavor, and yes it has great texture, but my favorite part about this recipe is that it is so easy to make.

| YIELD: 5 SERVINGS | PREP TIME: 20 MINUTES | COOKING TIME: 30 MINUTES |

wet ingredients

1 1/2 cups chick peas, cooked and drained
1/2 cup water
2 Tbsp olive oil
2 Tbsp apple juice
1 Tbsp soy sauce
1 Tbsp apple cider vinegar
2 tsp chicken-less base
1 tsp onion powder
1/2 tsp garlic powder
1/2 tsp poultry seasoning
1 tsp sugar
1/2 tsp salt

dry ingredients

1 cup Vital wheat gluten flour
1/4 cup nutritional yeast flakes
2 Tbsp rice flour

breading ingredients

1/2 cup bread crumbs
1/2 cup Panko
1/2 Tbsp basil

Watch the recipe here

directions

1. Preheat the oven to 400°F.
2. In a large bowl, smash the chickpeas with a fork.
3. Add the remaining wet ingredients, and mix well.
4. In another bowl, mix the dry ingredients together.
5. Combine the wet and the dry ingredients, and mix well. You will want to mix this for a good two minutes. This will provide some elasticity in the gluten.
6. Divide into 5 equal portions, and form into patties. This will have a soft texture, but try to keep it tight.
7. Bread the patties by lightly pressing into the breading mixture.
8. Place on a parchment lined sheet pan, and spray with a little olive oil spray.
9. Bake for a total of 30 minutes. 15 minutes on one side, then flip and lightly spray, then bake for another 15 minutes.
10. Best to cool on a wire rack.

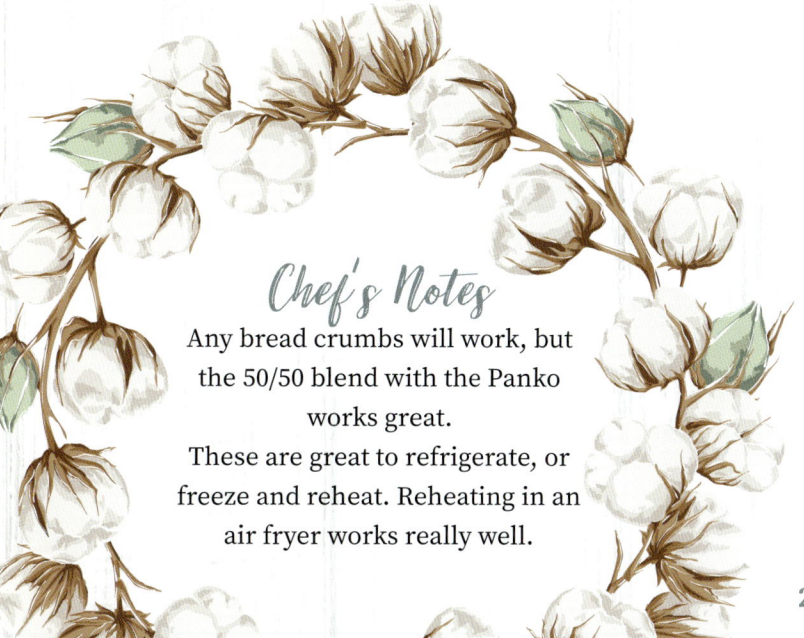

Chef's Notes
Any bread crumbs will work, but the 50/50 blend with the Panko works great.
These are great to refrigerate, or freeze and reheat. Reheating in an air fryer works really well.

BREAKFAST SAUSAGE

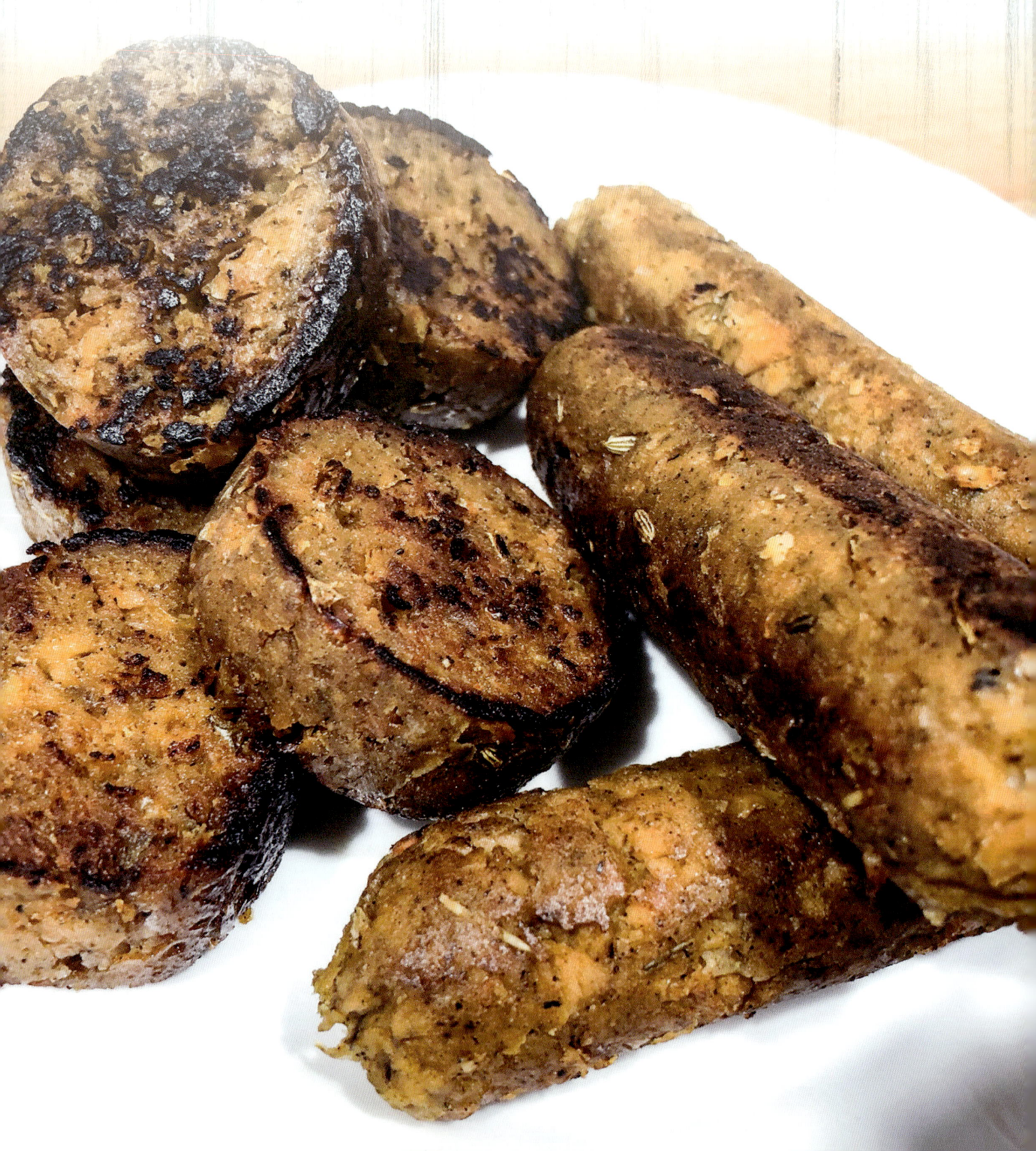

BREAKFAST SAUSAGE

This recipe is an old favorite that I started doing 15 years ago for large events.
And years later, I've never had to change a thing. You are going to love it!

| YIELD: 4 TO 6 SERVINGS | PREP TIME: 20 MINUTES | COOKING TIME: 30 MINUTES |

ingredients

1/2 cup TVP, soaked and drained
(textured vegetable protein)
1 cup cooked white kidney beans, rinsed
and drained
1 cup veggie broth
2 Tbsp olive oil
2 Tbsp Braggs Liquid Aminos
2 Tbsp maple syrup
1/4 cup nutritional yeast flakes
1 Tbsp sage
1 tsp paprika
1/2 tsp thyme
1/2 tsp rosemary
1/2 tsp whole fennel seed
Pinch cayenne
1 1/4 cup Vital wheat gluten flour

directions

1. Start by soaking the TVP for a few minutes, then drain it.
2. Mash beans and add all ingredients except wheat gluten. Mix well.
3. Add the wheat gluten. Mix very well and set aside.
4. Take about a golf ball size amount and wrap with foil just like a tootsie roll.
5. Place in oven water bath for 25 minutes at 350°F, or steam for 25 minutes.
6. Allow to cool a little and unwrap.
7. Reheat on the grill. Great for creating the grill markings.

Watch the recipe here

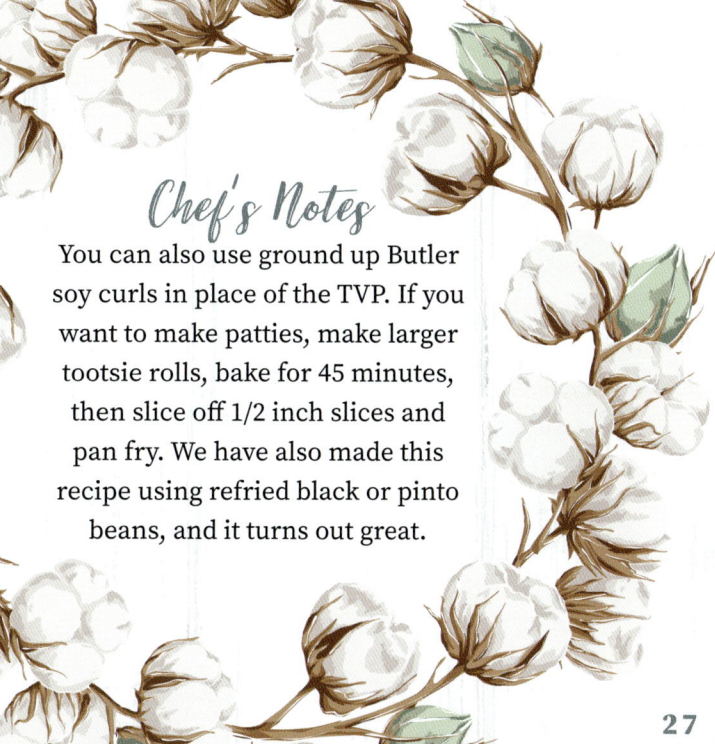

Chef's Notes

You can also use ground up Butler soy curls in place of the TVP. If you want to make patties, make larger tootsie rolls, bake for 45 minutes, then slice off 1/2 inch slices and pan fry. We have also made this recipe using refried black or pinto beans, and it turns out great.

27

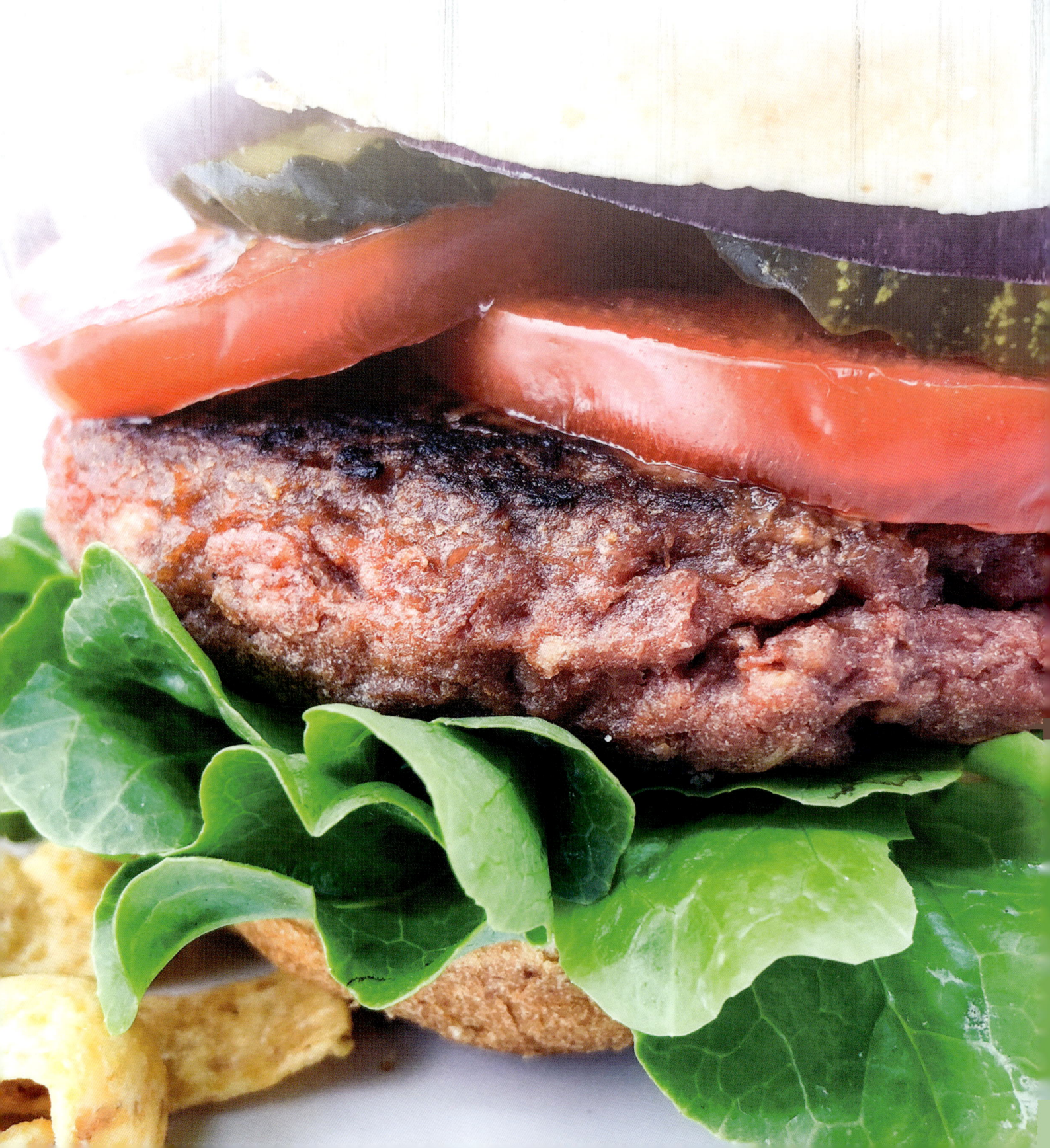

BUTLER BURGERS GLUTEN FREE

BUTLER BURGERS
GLUTEN FREE

If you're looking for a great burger, you've come to the right place. This is going to be an all time favorite. And it's good for you!

YIELD: 3 TO 6 SERVINGS	PREP TIME: 20 MINUTES	COOKING TIME: 10 MINUTES

dry ingredients

1 cup ground Butler Soy Curls
1/2 cup garbanzo bean flour
3 Tbsp nutritional yeast flakes
2 tsp onion powder
1 1/2 tsp beet powder
1 tsp cocoa powder
1 tsp garlic powder
1/2 tsp smoked paprika
1/2 tsp chili powder
1/2 tsp salt
1/2 tsp guar gum
1/2 tsp xanthan gum
1 Tbsp methylcellulose
(OR 2 Tbsp Tapioca starch)

wet ingredients

1 cup hot tap water
2 Tbsp soy sauce
2 Tbsp olive oil
1 tsp sugar
1/2 tsp liquid smoke

Watch the recipe here

directions

1. Mix dry ingredients.
2. Mix the wet ingredients.
3. Mix together, and allow to rest for 5 minutes.
4. Form into burgers. You can make 3 to 6 burgers.
5. Pan fry on medium to low heat. About 3 minutes per side.

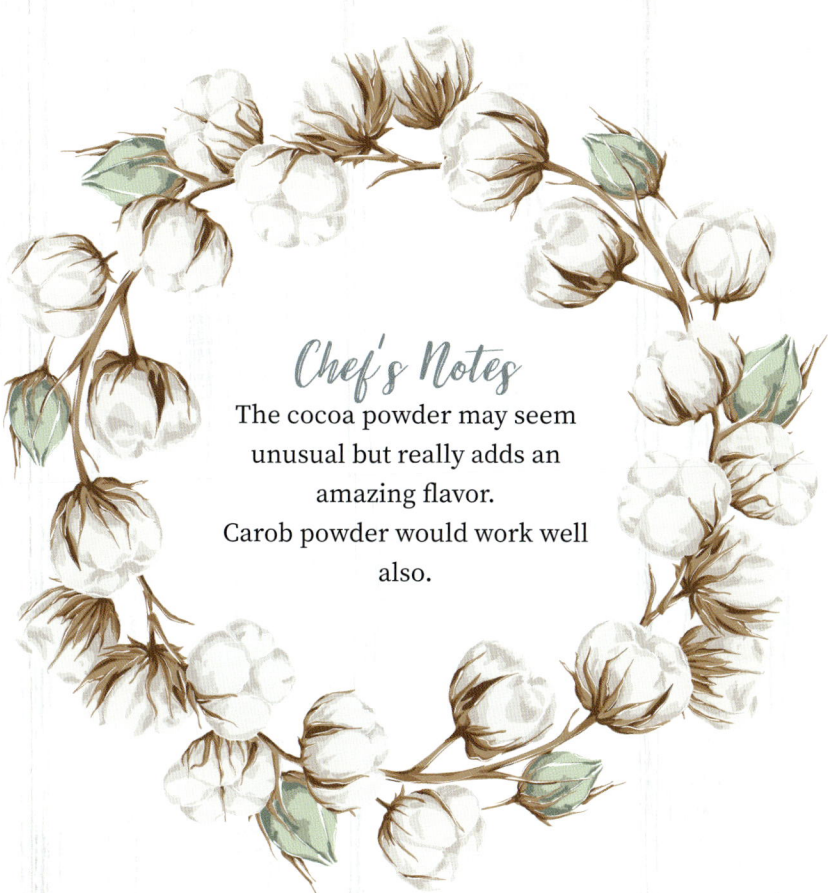

Chef's Notes
The cocoa powder may seem unusual but really adds an amazing flavor.
Carob powder would work well also.

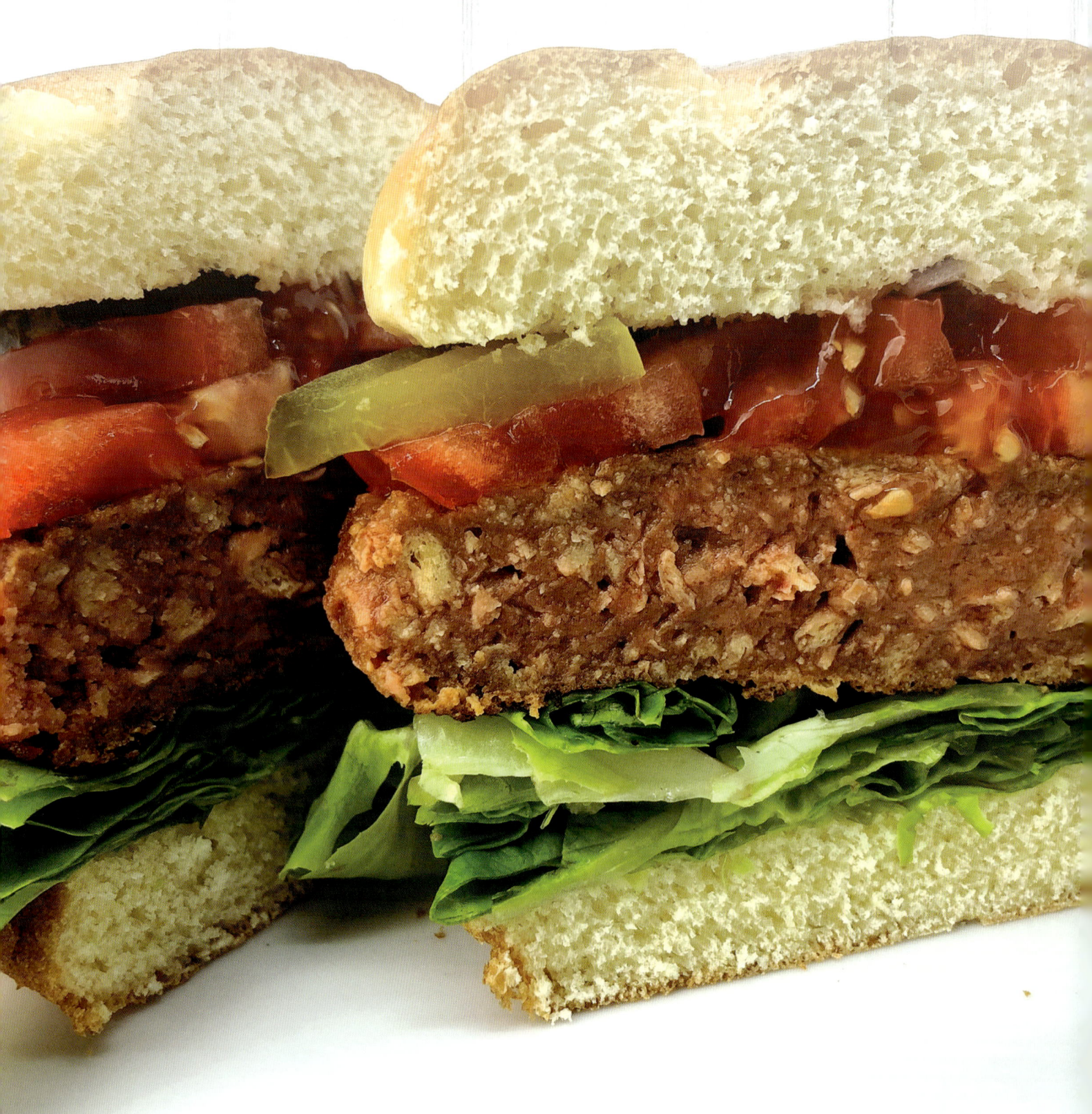

BUTLER BURGERS 4.0
GLUTEN FREE

This is the gourmet version of the original Butler Burger. By adding the jack fruit and mushrooms, the texture is really enhanced. The additional seasoning creates a simply delicious burger!

YIELD: 6 TO 8 SERVINGS	PREP TIME: 20 MINUTES	COOKING TIME: 10 MINUTES

dry ingredients

1 1/4 cups ground Butler Soy Curls
1/2 cup garbanzo bean flour
1/4 cup nutritional yeast flakes
1 Tbsp onion powder
1/2 Tbsp garlic powder
2 tsp beet powder
1 1/4 tsp cocoa powder
1 tsp smoked paprika
1 tsp chili powder
1 tsp salt
1 tsp guar gum
1 tsp xanthan gum
1 Tbsp + 1 tsp methylcellulose
OR 3 Tbsp Tapioca starch

wet ingredients

1 cup hot tap water
3 Tbsp soy sauce
1 tsp liquid smoke
1 1/2 tsp sugar
3 Tbsp olive oil
1/2 cup minced jack fruit
1/2 cup minced cooked mushrooms
(King oyster is best)

Watch the recipe here

directions

1. Mix dry ingredients.
2. Mix the wet ingredients.
3. Combine together, and allow to rest for 5 minutes.
4. Form into 6 to 8 burgers.
5. Pan fry on medium heat. About 3 minutes per side.

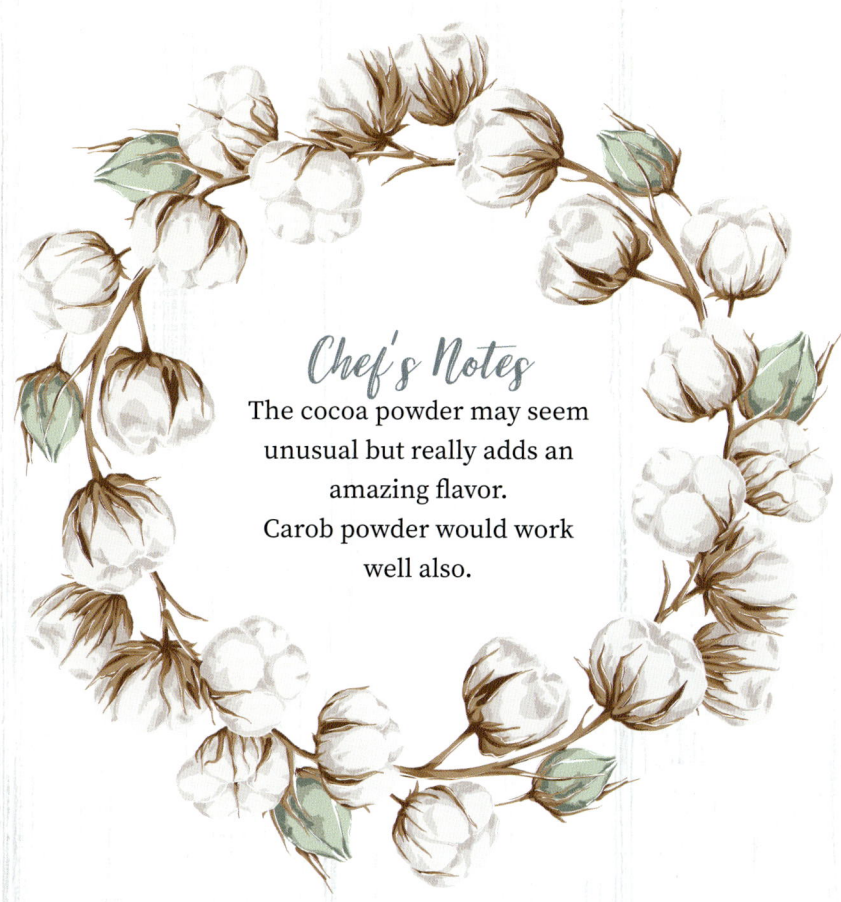

Chef's Notes
The cocoa powder may seem unusual but really adds an amazing flavor.
Carob powder would work well also.

CAVIAR

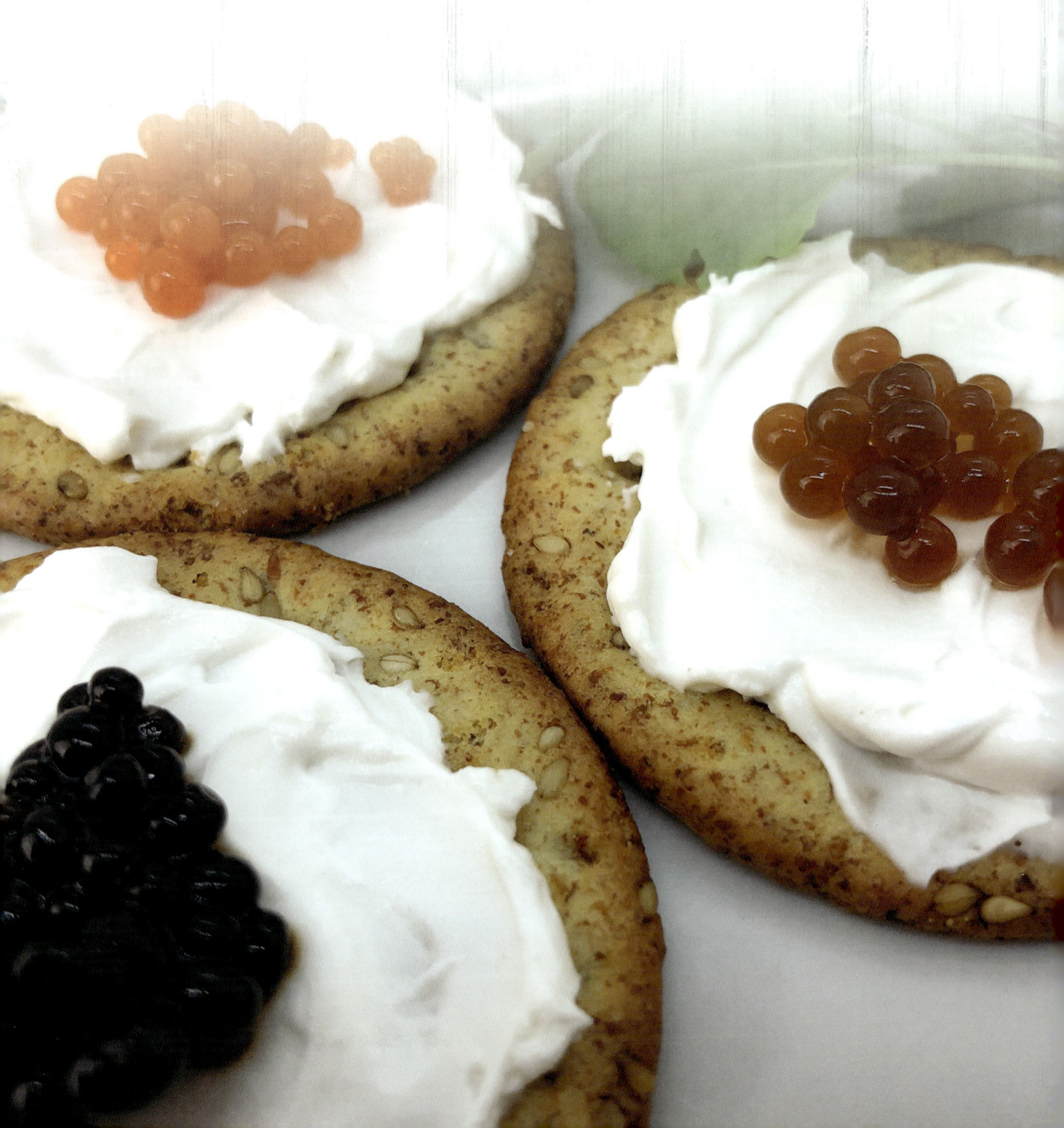

CAVIAR

Yes, a vegan imitation that is not going to cost you $12,000 a pound to produce it.
In fact, this will cost next to nothing and you probably already have the ingredients in your cupboard!
I have three different recipes for you: Original, Spicy and Teriyaki.

YIELD: 8 SERVINGS	PREP TIME: 5 MINUTES	COOKING TIME: 5 MINUTES

ORIGINAL (BELUGA)

ingredients

1/4 cup soy sauce
1/4 cup molasses
3/4 tsp Agar Agar powder

SPICY (SALMON)

ingredients

1/4 cup Sriracha Pepper Sauce
1/4 cup water
3/4 tsp Agar Agar powder

TERIYAKI (ALMAS)

ingredients

1/4 cup Teriyaki sauce
1/4 cup water
3/4 tsp Agar Agar powder

additional ingredients

Oil, vegetable or olive

directions

1. Chill a tall glass full of oil in the refrigerator overnight or for several hours, leaving about 2 inches of space at the top of the glass. This oil is just used to create the caviar beads. Any extra tall glass will work.
2. Mix the ingredients for the variation you are making. Bring to a boil and simmer for 2 minutes.
3. Transfer the mixture into a squeeze bottle and cool for a several minutes, but do not let this mixture get cold.
4. Slowly drip the mixture into the chilled oil. The size of the hole in the squeeze bottle will determine the size of the caviar. The cold oil will set the shape of the caviar.
5. After you are done dripping all the mixture into the oil, you will want to drain off the oil into a container through a mesh strainer. The oil can be reused for anything else.
6. Then take the caviar and rinse it in a bowl of cold water, to rinse the excess oil off.
7. Strain to collect the caviar and place into an airtight container for use.

Chef's Notes

This product has a very good shelf life when refrigerated. Re-rinse the caviar if unused for a couple days. This will keep it from bleeding into your finished creation. Serve on a cracker with vegan cream cheese.

Watch the recipe here

33

CHICKEN DRUMSTICKS BBQ STYLE

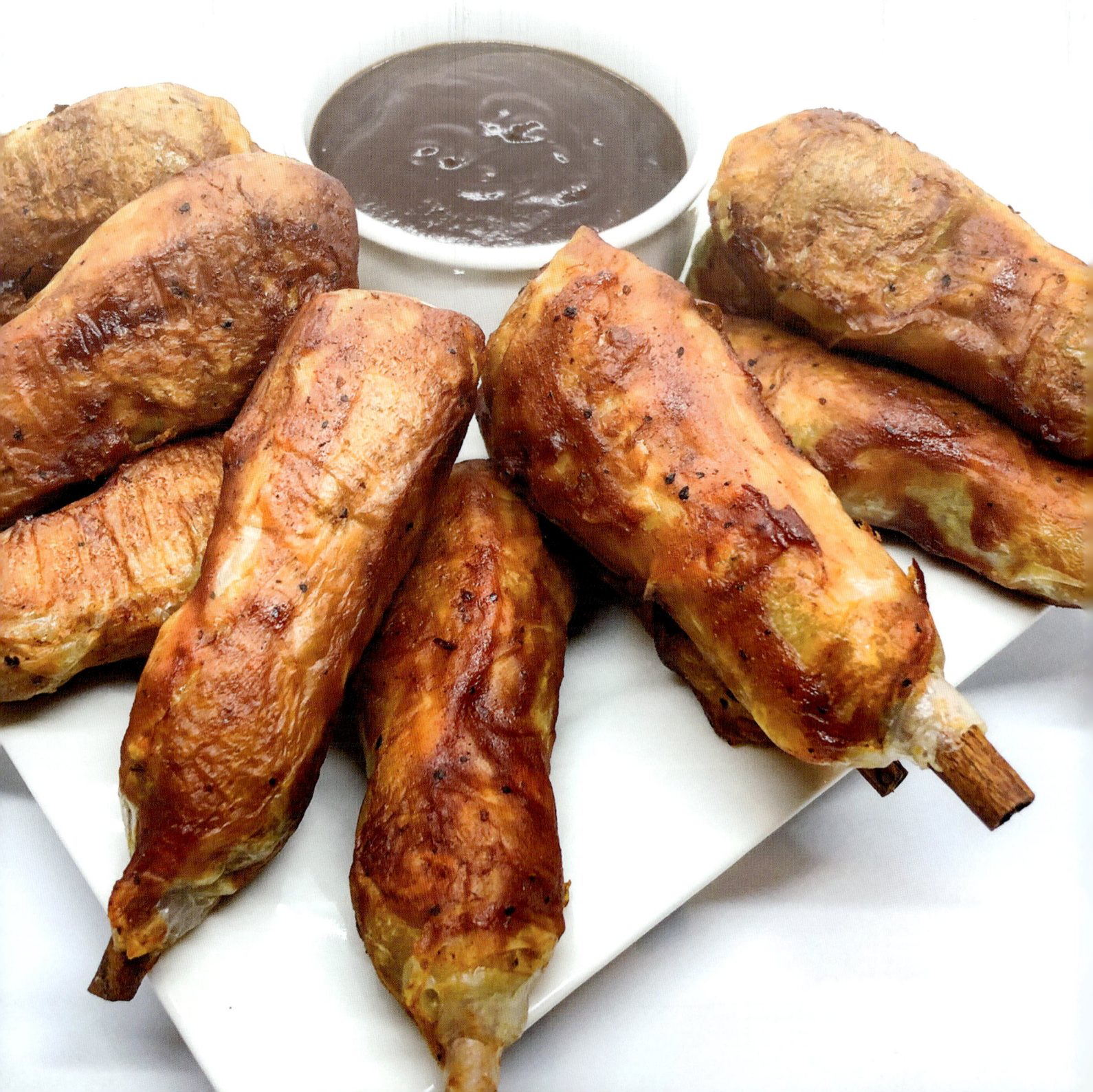

CHICKEN DRUMSTICKS
BBQ STYLE

YIELD: 12 DRUMSTICKS	PREP TIME: 20 MINUTES	COOKING TIME: 1.3 HOURS

wet ingredients

2 cans jack fruit (cooked and squeeze drained)
1 1/2 cup chick peas, cooked and drained
1/4 cup water
1/4 cup BBQ sauce
2 Tbsp olive oil
2 Tbsp apple juice
1 Tbsp chicken-less base
1 Tbsp soy sauce
1 Tbsp apple cider vinegar
2 tsp onion powder
1 tsp garlic powder
1 tsp poultry seasoning
1 tsp sugar
1/2 tsp salt

dry ingredients

3/4 cup Vital wheat gluten flour
1/2 cup nutritional yeast flakes
2 Tbsp rice flour

additional ingredients

12 sugar cane swizzle sticks, or popsicle sticks
12 small sheets of rice paper
1/2 cup BBQ sauce for splashing

FAMOUS SEASONED FLOUR

1 cups unbleached all-purpose flour
2 Tbsp smoked paprika
3/4 Tbsp white pepper
1/2 Tbsp sea salt
1/2 Tbsp onion powder
1/2 Tbsp garlic powder
1/2 Tbsp ginger
1/2 Tbsp celery salt
1/2 Tbsp dried mustard
1/2 tsp dried oregano
1/4 Tbsp thyme
1/4 Tbsp basil

directions

1. Boil off the jack fruit for 30 minutes, then cool.
2. Preheat oven to 375°F.
3. Squeeze the jack fruit to remove as much moisture as possible, and then make sure it is well shredded.
4. Smash the chick peas with a fork.
5. Combine all the wet ingredients and mix well.
6. In a separate bowl, mix the dry ingredients.
7. Combine the wet and dry ingredients. Make sure to knead for a good three minutes in order to create some elasticity in the gluten.
8. Divide the dough into 12 equal portions.
9. Wrap each portion with rice paper. You will want to form the portion into the look of a drumstick with the cinnamon stick in the center as the bone.
10. The rice paper will need to be wet in order to wrap around the drumstick. Soak on a cutting board in warm water until softened. Then wrap the rice paper around the meat as tight as possible.
11. Splash the drumsticks with BBQ sauce and place on a parchment lined sheet pan.
12. In the oven, use the middle rack, and bake for 45 minutes. Every 15 minutes, you are going to rub with more bbq sauce and rotate. They should have a nice browned color and texture.

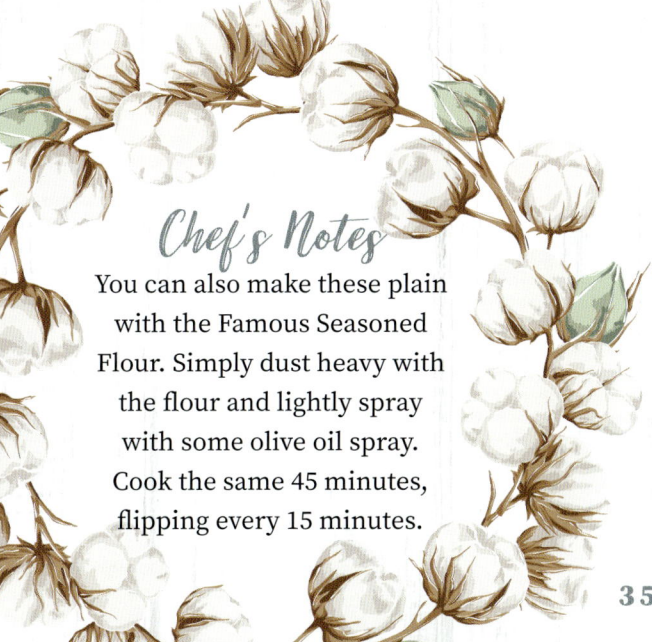

Chef's Notes
You can also make these plain with the Famous Seasoned Flour. Simply dust heavy with the flour and lightly spray with some olive oil spray. Cook the same 45 minutes, flipping every 15 minutes.

Watch the recipe here

CHICKEN FRIED STEAK

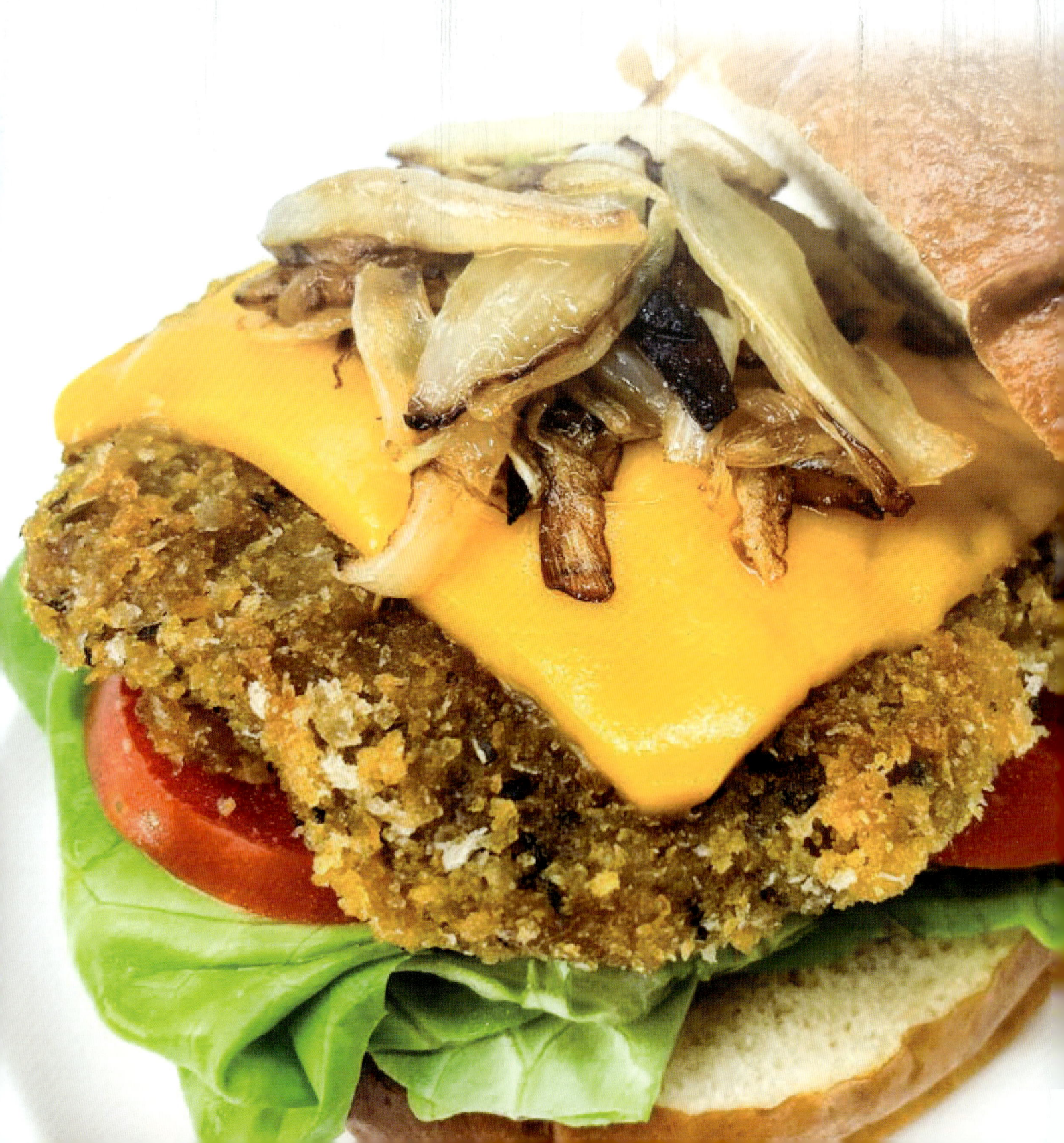

CHICKEN FRIED STEAK

This is an old favorite that we have done many times for 1,000 people or more. It is one of the most delicious vegan meat recipes I have ever had. Well worth the time it takes to make.

YIELD: 4 TO 6 SERVINGS	PREP TIME: 20 MINUTES	COOKING TIME: 30 MINUTES

dry ingredients

1 1/2 cups Vital wheat gluten flour

1/2 cup rice flour

wet ingredients

2 cups water

6 Tbsp soy sauce or Braggs Liquid Aminos

2 Tbsp granulated garlic

2 Tbsp powdered onion

2 Tbsp beef-less base

additional ingredients

1/2 package tofu (any style works)

1 cup soy milk

2 cups bread crumbs

2 cups flour

directions

1. Preheat oven to 350°F.

2. Mix the wet ingredients well so that the beef-less base is dissolved.

3. Then add the mixed dry ingredients and mix well.

4. Form into patties and place on parchment lined sheet pans.

5. Cook steaks for 7 to 10 minutes or more on each side. It all depends on how thick you make them. When done, they should be fully cooked in the inside, and not gooey. But don't over cook them into cardboard.

6. For the breading process, you will want to blend the tofu and milk into a thick egg like substitute.

7. Start the breading with the flour first, then the tofu mixture, then the bread crumbs.

8. Pan fry the steaks with a little olive oil until golden brown on both sides.

Chef's Notes

If you have plain bread crumbs add some Italian seasoning and salt. Make big batches, because these freeze well.

Watch the recipe here

CORNED BEEF BRISKET GLUTEN FREE

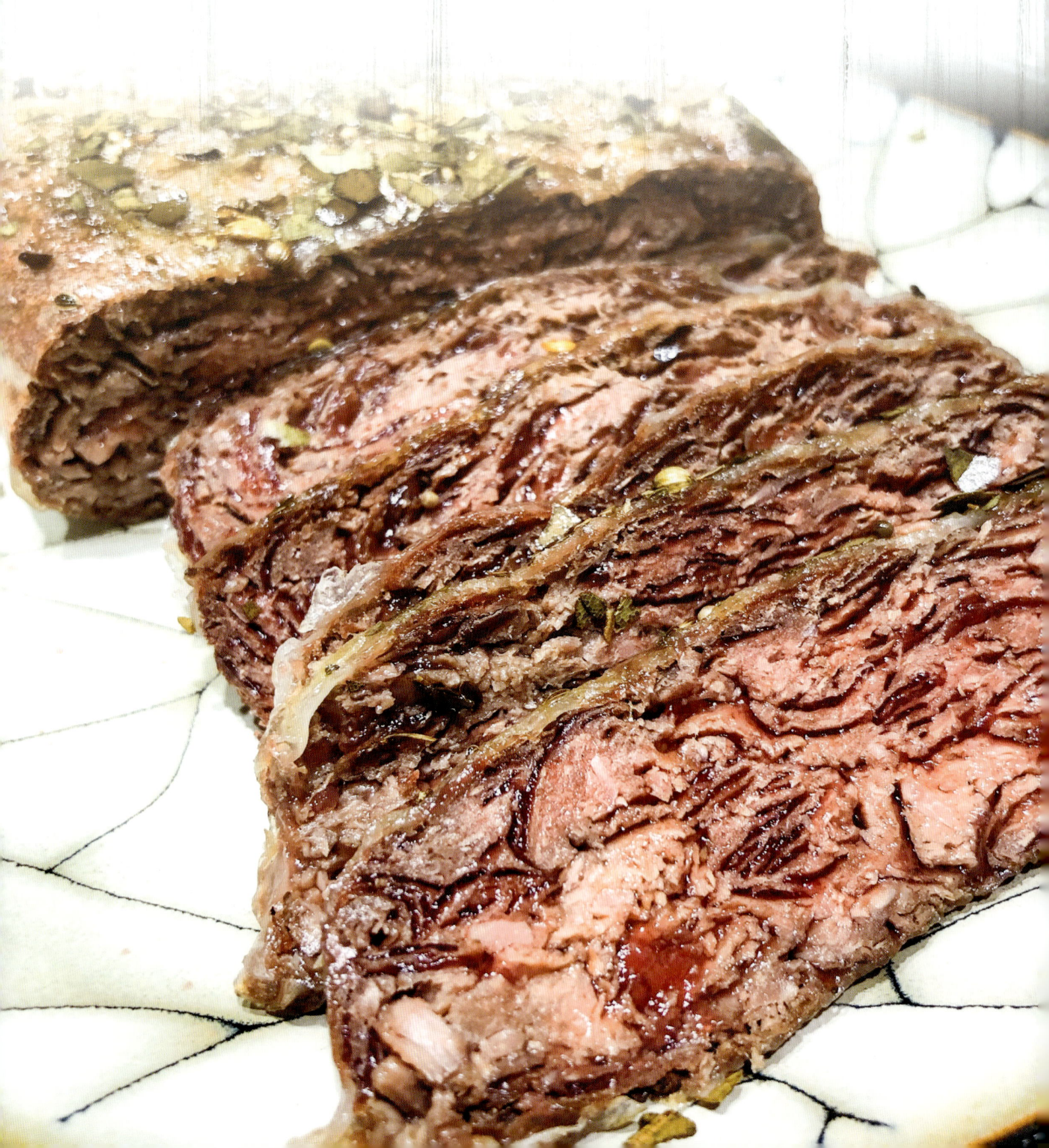

CORNED BEEF BRISKET
GLUTEN FREE

This recipe is a dream come true for corned beef lovers. It has a unique flavor. And the texture meets my requirements for being much like the real thing. Serve this with cabbage, new potatoes and carrots, and you'll feel right at home... in Ireland. And yes, it's gluten free.

YIELD: 8 SERVINGS	PREP TIME: 25 MINUTES	COOKING TIME: 1.75 HOURS

wet ingredients

3 cans jack fruit, drained
3 cups water
1 cup apple juice
1/3 cup apple cider vinegar
1/3 cup pickling spice
2 Tbsp chicken base
2 Tbsp liquid smoke
2 tsp salt

dry ingredients

1 cup chickpea flour
1/4 cup rice flour
1/4 cup tapioca flour
4 Tbsp beet powder
2 Tbsp xanthan gum
5 sheets rice paper blended into small pieces.

additional items

4 sheets rice paper
Oil for frying
Additional pickling spice for baking time

Watch the recipe here

directions

1. Simmer the wet ingredients for 30 minutes, just under a boil.
2. Allow to cool in the juice.
3. Drain the jack fruit, reserving only 3/4 cup of the juice that it was cooked in.
4. Mash the jack fruit into a shredded 'meat'.
5. Blend the first 5 rice paper sheets into small pieces, not powder.
6. Mix the rice paper with all the dry ingredients.
7. Mix together with the wet ingredients.
8. Wrap with the 4 whole rice paper sheets. You will want watch the video on this part. The rice paper needs to be wet in order to make it stretch. On a wet cutting board, taking two at a time and slightly overlapped, you will place the meat on top and then wrap, connecting the rice paper. Repeat the process on the other side.
9. Then pan fry the brisket in a hot oiled pan. This will seal the rice paper.
10. On a parchment lined sheet pan, sprinkle about 2 Tbsp of pickling spice, then place the brisket on the spices. Sprinkle a little more pickling spice on the top.
11. You will want to bake this at 350°F for about 75 minutes. Flip over half way through the cooking process.
12. Allow to cool, or refrigerate overnight, then slice. Reheat when ready to serve.

CRAB CAKES

CRAB CAKES

This recipe great to use for either crab cakes or for seafood croquets.
It just depends what way you chose to shape them.

YIELD: 12 CRAB CAKES	PREP TIME: 25 MINUTES	COOKING TIME: 45 MINUTES

ingredients

2 cans jackfruit, drained
2 cans cannellini beans, rinsed and drained
1/4 cup chopped red bell pepper
1/4 cup chopped onions
1/4 cup vegan mayo
1 tsp onion powder
1 tsp garlic powder
1 tsp salt
1 tsp old bay seasoning
1/2 tsp mustard powder
2 tsp dulse powder (red seaweed powder)
1 pack roasted seaweed sheets
1 lemon, juiced
1/4 cup ground flax seed mixed
with 1/4 cup hot water

breadcrumb mixture

3 cups Panko bread crumbs
3 Tbsp nutritional yeast flakes
1 Tbsp parsley flakes

directions

1. Preheat oven to 425°F.
2. In a food processor, pulse together the jackfruit, beans, and seaweed. Don't over blend, you want a lot of flakiness from the jackfruit.
3. Mix together the spices.
4. Add the jackfruit mixture, pepper, onion, ground flax seed, vegan mayo, and lemon. Hand mix well.
5. Form into crab cake shapes and carefully bread in the breadcrumb mixture.
6. Place the crab cakes on a parchment paper lined sheet pan.
7. Spray with a little olive oil spray.
8. Bake for 45 minutes. 20 minutes on one side, then flip and spray with olive oil and cook for another 20 to 25 minutes. They should be golden brown.

Watch the recipe here

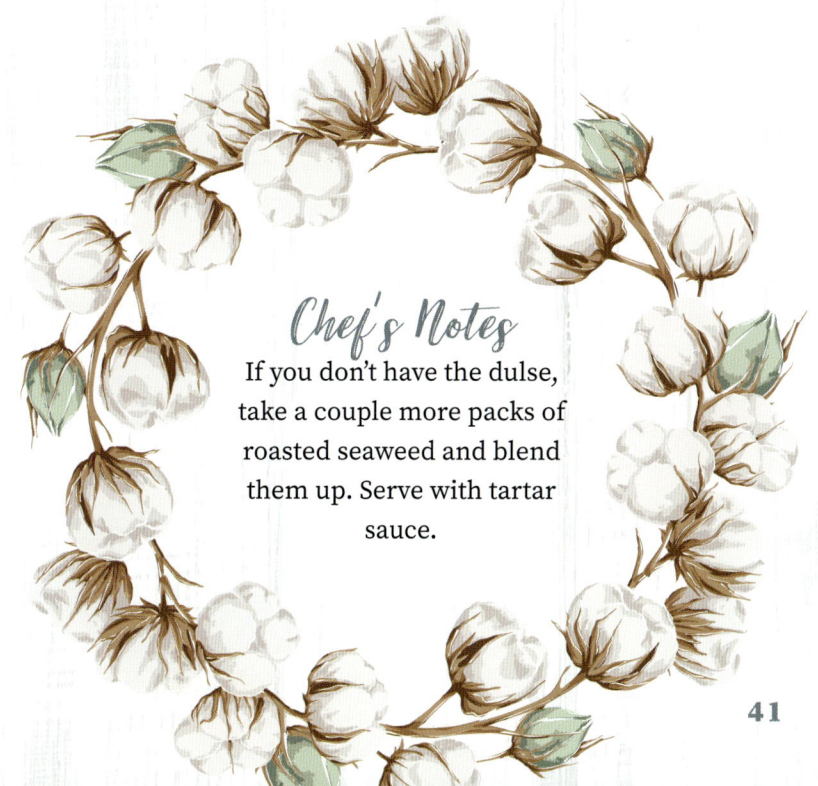

Chef's Notes

If you don't have the dulse, take a couple more packs of roasted seaweed and blend them up. Serve with tartar sauce.

CROCKPOT HAM

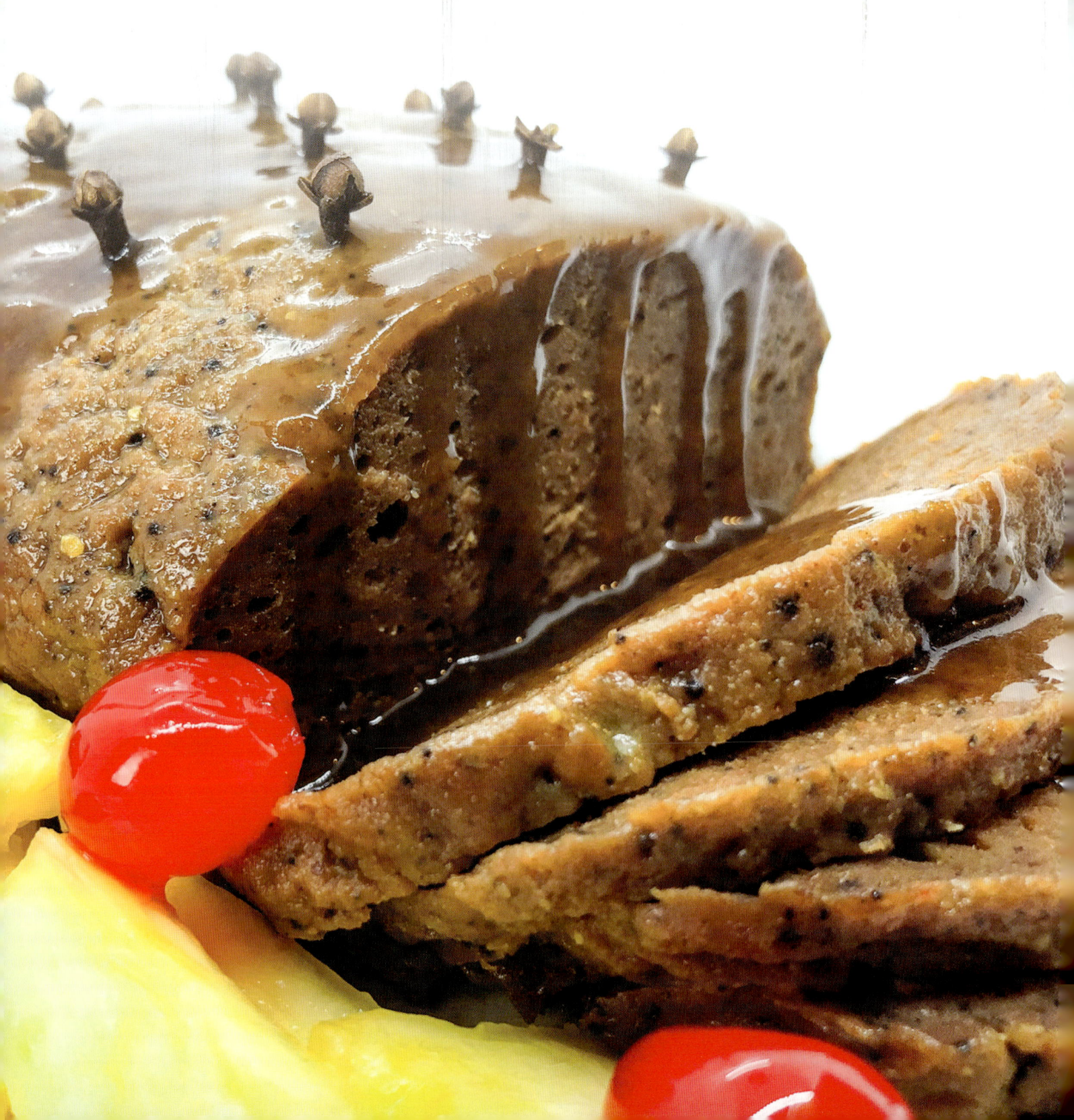

CROCKPOT HAM

This recipe is a little darker in color from the traditional ham; so it gets to keep its own identity. The flavor is absolutely amazing, and I'm glad that I didn't sacrifice flavor for color.

YIELD: 10+ SERVINGS	PREP TIME: 20 MINUTES	COOKING TIME: 4 HOURS

wet ingredients

1 cup water
1 cup tomato sauce
1/2 cup pineapple juice
2 Tbsp tomato paste
2 Tbsp soy sauce
2 Tbsp veggie base
2 Tbsp maple syrup
2 Tbsp liquid smoke
2 Tbsp onion powder
1 Tbsp garlic
1 Tbsp smoked paprika
1/2 tsp ground cloves
1/2 tsp salt
1/4 tsp white pepper

dry ingredients

3 cups Vital wheat gluten flour
1/2 cup rice flour
1/4 cup tapioca flour

glaze

1/2 cup brown sugar
1/4 cup pineapple juice
2 Tbsp spicy brown mustard
1 Tbsp molasses
2 Tbsp butter

Watch the recipe here

directions

1. Mix wet ingredients
2. In a separate bowl, mix the dry ingredients.
3. Combine the wet and dry and mix well, forming into a loaf-like shape.
4. In a large crockpot you will cook the 'ham' for 2 hours on low, and then 2 hours on high. I suggest watching the video to see how to set up the crockpot. I make a little foil ring around the bottom of the crockpot, then place the 'ham' in parchment paper before putting in the crockpot. Then I add one cup of water on the outside of the parchment paper.
5. After cooking, place in a baking casserole dish and cover with the well mixed glaze.
6. Cook for 20 to 30 minutes at 350 °F. You will see a nice browning.
7. Allow to cool before cutting to serve, or chill overnight and slice for your deli meat.

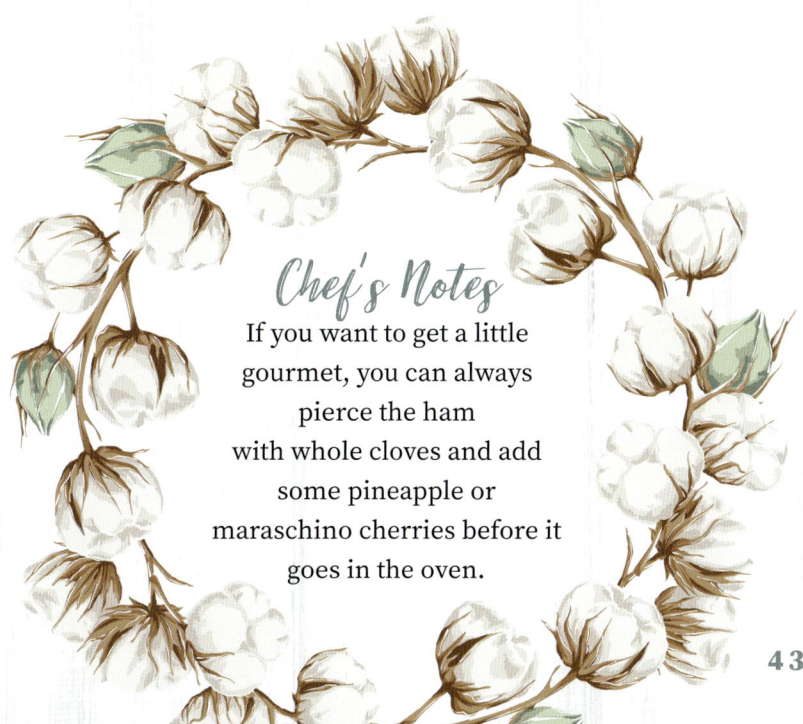

Chef's Notes
If you want to get a little gourmet, you can always pierce the ham with whole cloves and add some pineapple or maraschino cherries before it goes in the oven.

EGGPLANT BACON

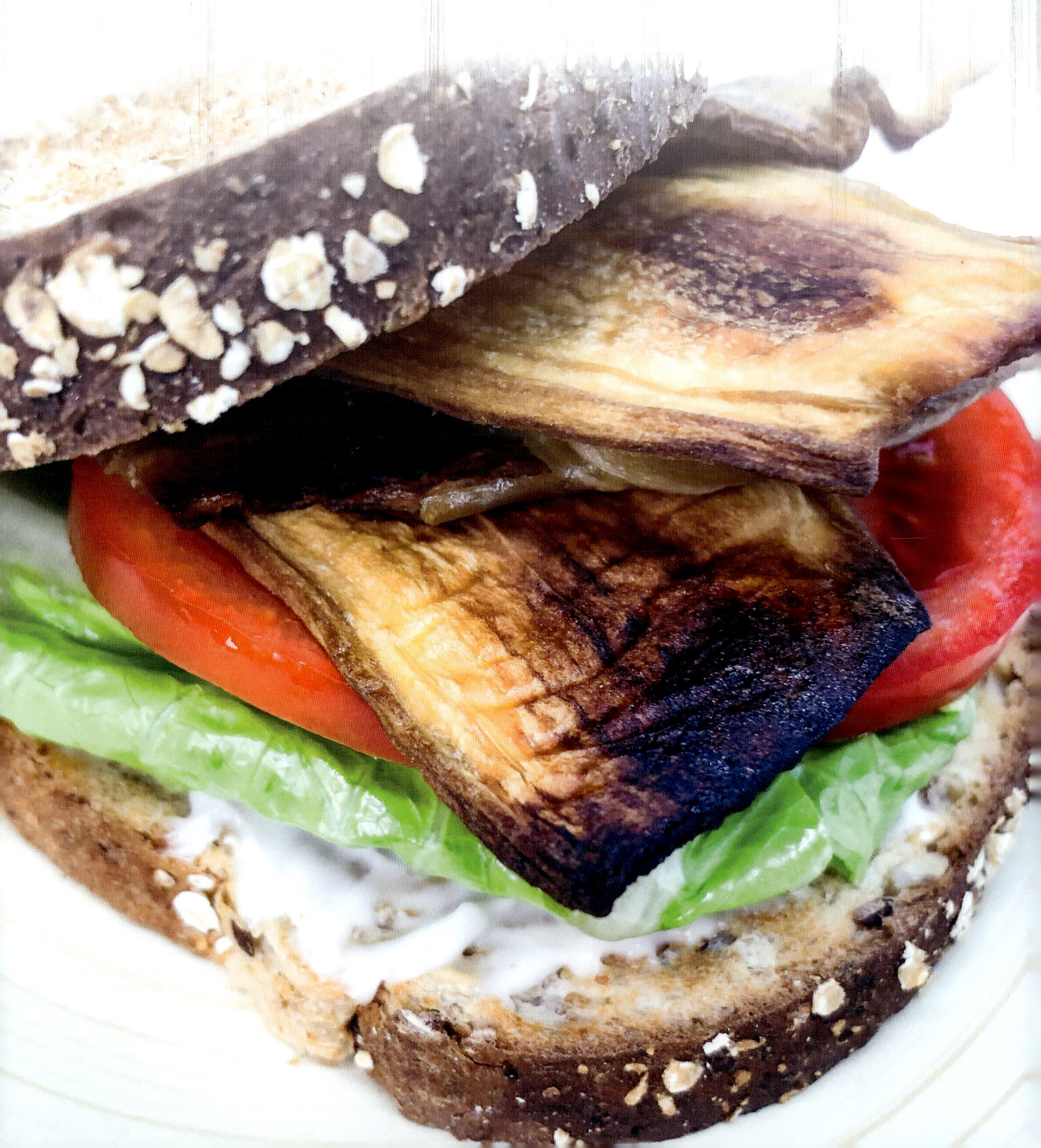

EGGPLANT BACON

| YIELD: 4 SERVINGS | PREP TIME: 20 MINUTES | COOKING TIME: 45 MINUTES |

ingredients

1 eggplant
1/4 cup maple syrup
1 Tbsp coconut oil
1 tsp liquid smoke
2 tsp salt

directions

1. Preheat oven to 350°F.
2. Peel the eggplant first, then slice the eggplant thin about 1/8 inch thick.
3. Salt the eggplant, and set aside for 30 minutes. This will allow the slices to sweat, and remove a lot of moisture.
4. Create a marinade with the remaining ingredients.
5. Lay out the eggplant on a parchment paper lined sheet pan. Depending how thin your slices are, you might need 2 pans.
6. Splash both sides of eggplant with the marinade.
7. Bake at 350°F for about 40 minutes or until crisp, flipping over half way through the process.
8. Allow to dry/cool on paper towels to absorb moisture.

Chef's Notes

This is my favorite bacon for an ELT Sandwich (*Eggplant, Lettuce, Tomato*).
You can also crunch it up and use it for bacon toppings and garnishing.

Watch the recipe here

EGGPLANT PHILLY

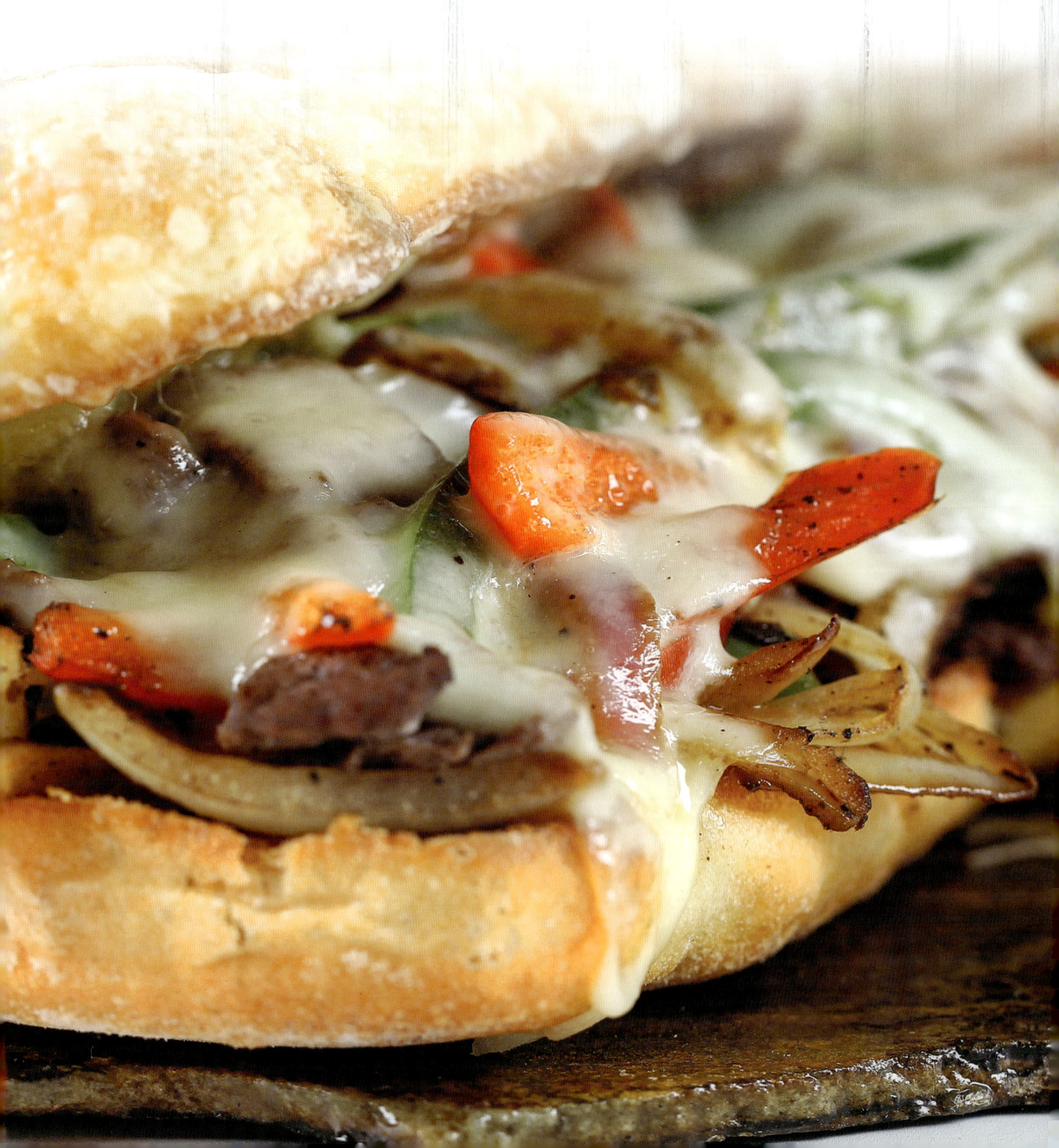

EGGPLANT PHILLY

YIELD: 2 TO 3 SERVINGS	PREP TIME: 15 MINUTES	COOKING TIME: 15 MINUTES

ingredients

1 eggplant
1 onion, slivered
1 red bell pepper, sliced
hoagie rolls
oil for sautéing
Vegan Mozzarella cheese

directions

1. Preheat the oven to 425°F.
2. Start by sautéing the onions and bell peppers.
3. Remove the skin from the eggplant and slice into very thin slices.
4. Add to the sautéd vegetables.
5. Sauté until everything is well cooked.
6. Take the hoagie rolls and toast in the oven a bit, only about 1 to two minutes.
7. Place the sautéed eggplant into the hoagies. Make sure it's not soggy. If so place on a paper towel for a minute to absorb the moisture.
8. Top with the vegan cheese.
9. Place back in the oven just until cheese is melted, for a couple minutes.

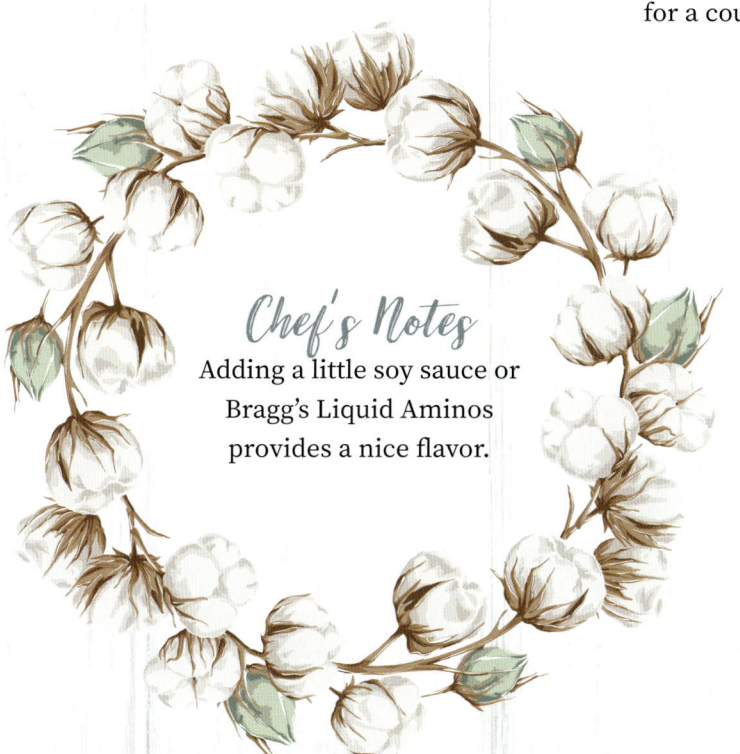

Chef's Notes
Adding a little soy sauce or Bragg's Liquid Aminos provides a nice flavor.

Watch the recipe here

FRIED BOLOGNA

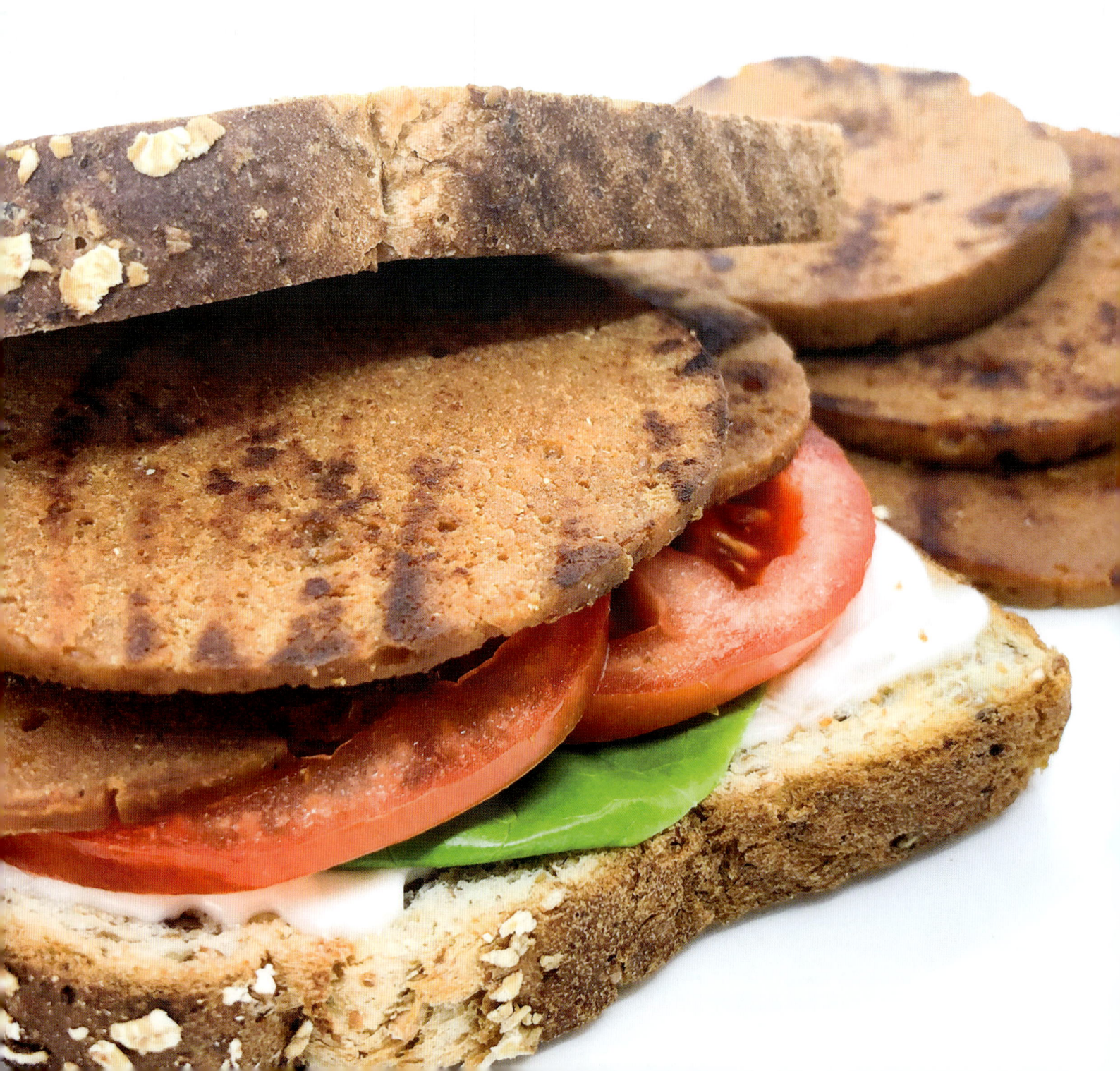

FRIED BOLOGNA

This recipe will take some of you back to childhood where fried bologna was a staple in many homes. Great for slicing in sandwiches and dicing for salads. And when you fry it, you will get an amazing meat substitute that will inspire you to make this a staple in your refrigerator.

YIELD: 10+ SERVINGS	PREP TIME: 15 MINUTES	COOKING TIME: 1.6 HOURS

wet ingredients

2 cups water
3/4 cup raw cashews
1/2 cup tomato sauce
1/4 cup nutritional yeast flakes
2 Tbsp beef-less base
2 Tbsp ground coriander
2 Tbsp sugar
2 Tbsp onion powder
1 Tbsp garlic powder
1 Tbsp paprika, smoked
1 Tbsp sea salt
1 tsp celery seed
1 tsp smoke

dry ingredients

2 cups Vital wheat gluten flour
2 Tbsp whole wheat flour
1/4 cup tapioca flour
1/4 cup rice flour

additional ingredients

Oil for frying

Watch the recipe here

directions

1. Preheat oven to 325°F.
2. Blend the wet ingredients until very smooth.
3. In a large bowl, mix the dry ingredients.
4. Combine the two ingredients and mix well.
5. Do a tootsie roll wrap first with parchment paper, and then twice with foil.
6. Bake for 1 1/2 hours.
7. Chill in fridge overnight. Then it's ready to unwrap and slice and pan fry with a little coconut oil.

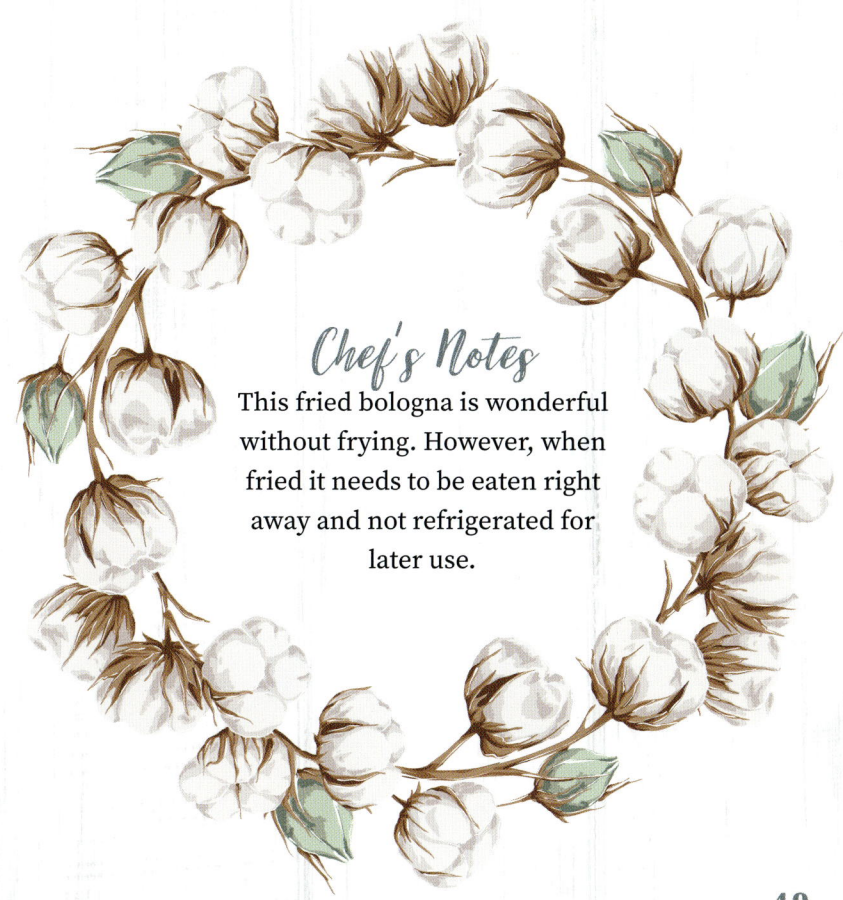

Chef's Notes

This fried bologna is wonderful without frying. However, when fried it needs to be eaten right away and not refrigerated for later use.

HOT DOGS GLUTEN FREE

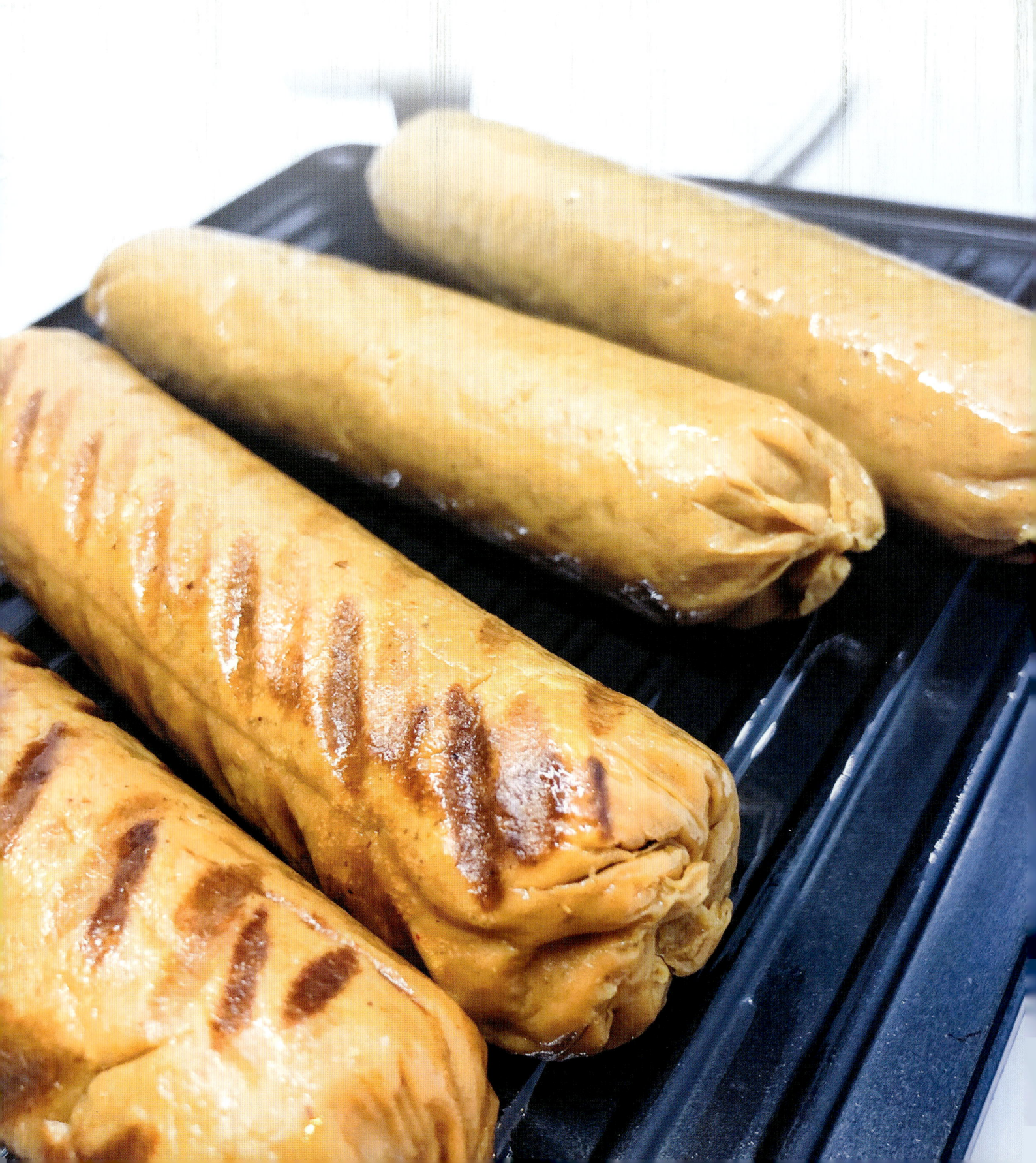

HOT DOGS
GLUTEN FREE

That's right - Gluten free! We have done the impossible. I have attempted to create a hot dog recipe dozens of times, with nothing that would even come close to the quality that I demand from my recipes. But through each failure, I learned something that I could use in the final product.
And eventually landed on the perfect gluten free hot dog. This is a really simple recipe to follow.

YIELD: 6 SERVINGS	PREP TIME: 15 MINUTES	COOKING TIME: 30 MINUTES

wet ingredients

1 King oyster mushroom, chopped
1 can Cannelloni beans, rinsed and drained
1/4 cup nutritional yeast flakes
3 Tbsp spicy brown mustard
3 Tbsp brown sugar
2 Tbsp tomato paste
2 Tbsp miso paste
2 Tbsp olive oil
2 Tbsp coriander
2 Tbsp onion powder
1 Tbsp garlic powder
1 Tbsp salt
1 tsp liquid smoke
1 tsp smoked paprika

dry ingredients

3/4 cup rice flour (112 g)
1 Tbsp xanthan gum

directions

1. Blend wet ingredients in food processor until very smooth.
2. Mix dry ingredients.
3. Combine the wet and dry and hand mix until well incorporated.
4. Divide into 6 equal portions.
5. Wrap like tootsie rolls in both parchment paper and then foil.
6. Steam for 30 minutes.
7. Allow to cool in refrigerator until cold.
8. Unwrap and they are ready to reheat and serve.

Watch the recipe here

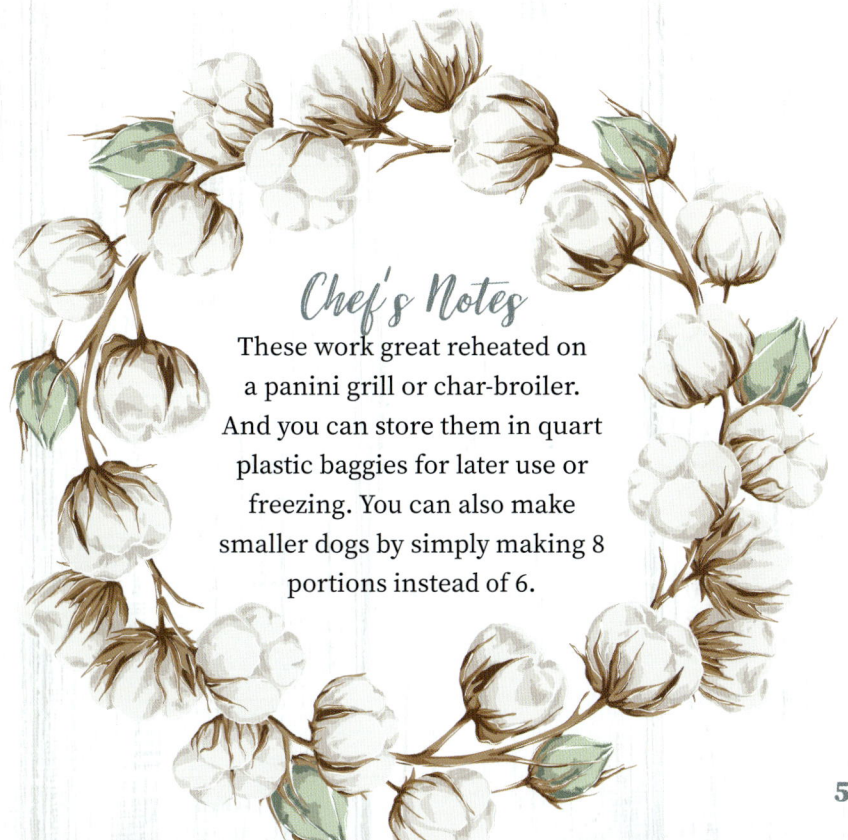

Chef's Notes

These work great reheated on a panini grill or char-broiler. And you can store them in quart plastic baggies for later use or freezing. You can also make smaller dogs by simply making 8 portions instead of 6.

ITALIAN SAUSAGE

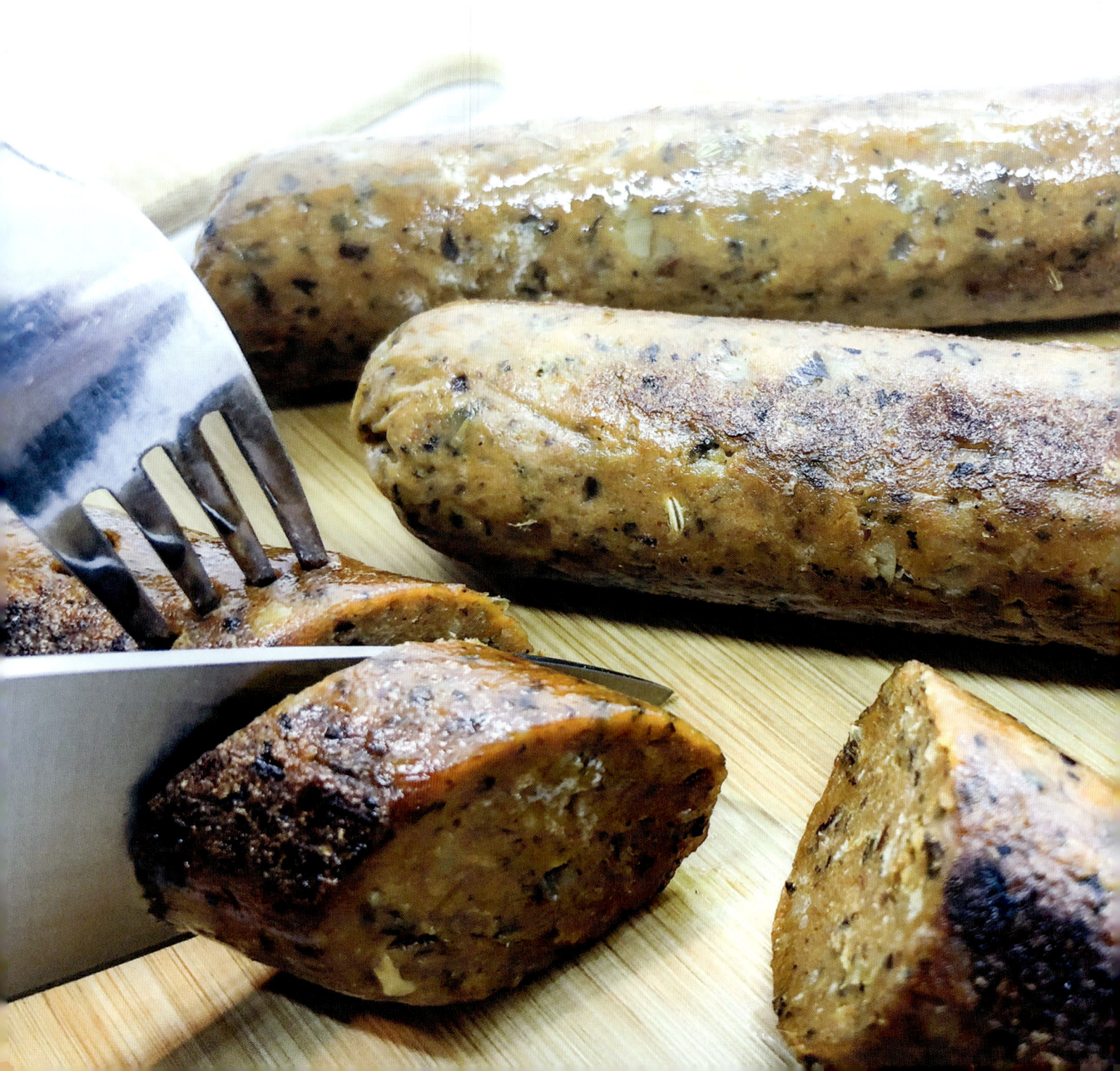

ITALIAN SAUSAGE

If you are looking to capture the likeness of a true Italian sausage, this is it. We have created the perfect combination of flavor and texture, but with a fraction of the fat that those Italian sausages normally have.

YIELD: 6 SERVINGS	PREP TIME: 15 MINUTES	COOKING TIME: 45 MINUTES

wet ingredients

3/4 cup water
2 Tbsp soy sauce
2 Tbsp garlic minced
2 Tbsp olive oil
2 Tbsp tomato paste
2 tsp liquid smoke
1 Tbsp basil
2 tsp oregano
1 Tbsp sugar
1 tsp fennel seeds
1 tsp thyme
1 tsp salt
1/2 tsp chili powder

dry ingredients

1 cup Vital wheat gluten flour
1 tsp smoked paprika
1 Tbsp garbanzo bean flour
1 Tbsp minced onions
2 Tbsp onion powder
2 tsp garlic powder

for hot italian

Use 1 Tbsp smoked paprika, and add 1/2 tsp red pepper flakes to the wet ingredients.

directions

1. Hand whip the wet ingredients together.
2. In a separate bowl, mix the dry ingredients.
3. Combine the wet with the dry and mix well
4. Divide into 4 portions, and tootsie roll wrap with parchment paper and then foil.
5. Steam for 45 minutes.
6. While still in foil, cool in fridge overnight.
7. Unwrap and they are ready to reheat and serve.

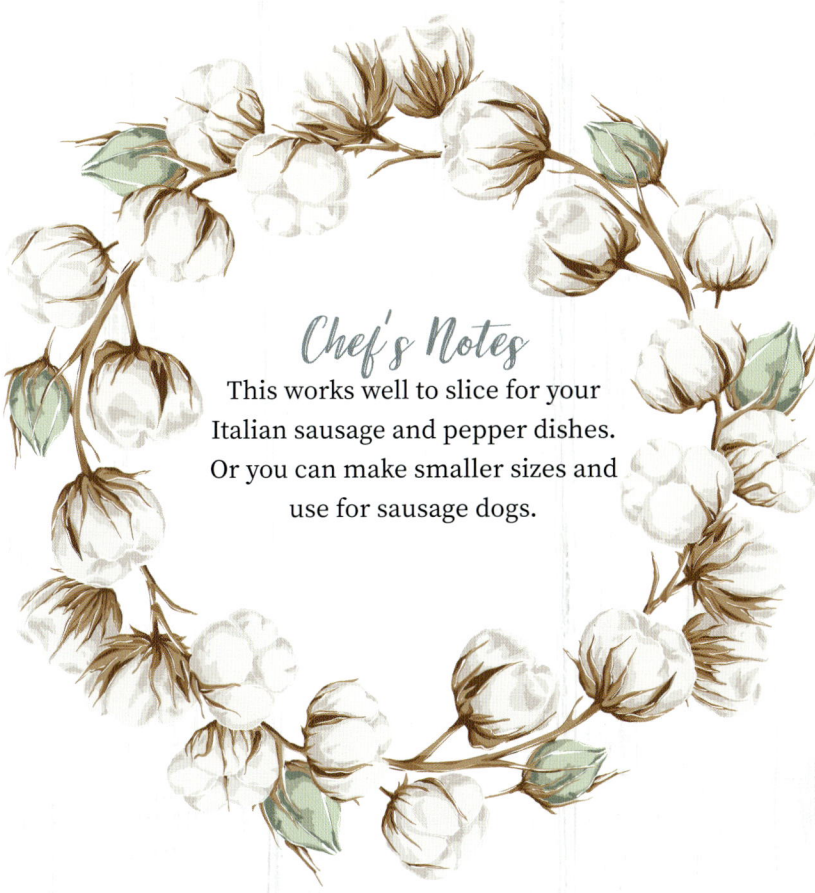

Chef's Notes

This works well to slice for your Italian sausage and pepper dishes. Or you can make smaller sizes and use for sausage dogs.

Watch the recipe here

ITALIAN SAUSAGE GLUTEN FREE

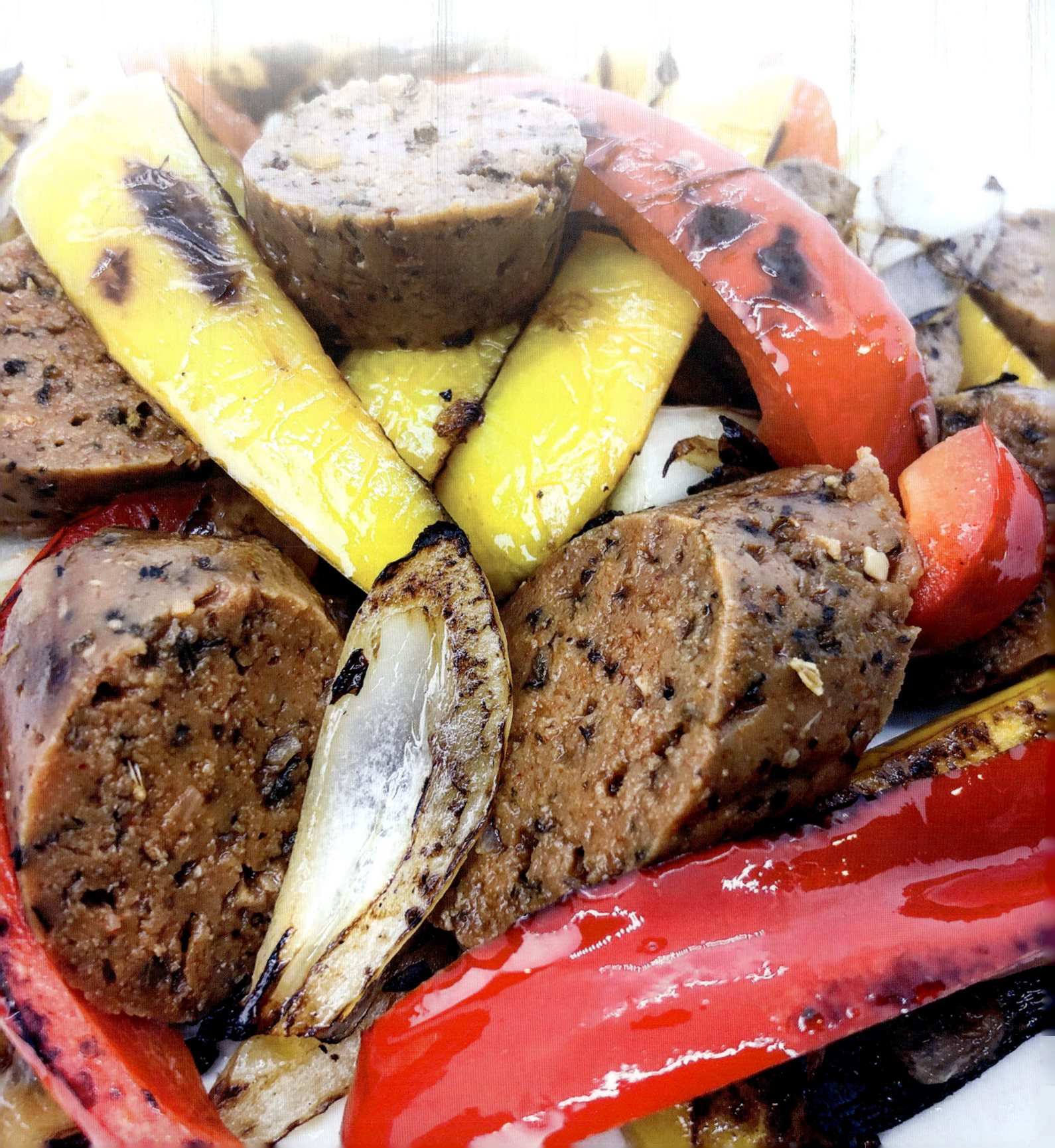

ITALIAN SAUSAGE
GLUTEN FREE

*Here is another wonderful vegan, gluten free recipe. It is great for a sausage dog,
or use it for slicing and make great Italian sausage dishes.*

YIELD: 4 TO 6 SERVINGS	PREP TIME: 15 MINUTES	COOKING TIME: 30 MINUTES

wet ingredients

1 - 6.5 oz can of mushrooms, drained
1 - 15 oz can black eyed peas, rinsed and drained
1/4 cup nutritional yeast flakes
2 Tbsp olive oil
2 Tbsp Vegan Worcestershire sauce
1 Tbsp soy sauce
1 Tbsp tomato paste
1 Tbsp garlic, minced
2 Tbsp onion powder
1 Tbsp smoked paprika
2 tsp salt
1 tsp oregano
1 tsp basil
1tsp thyme
1 tsp fennel seeds
1/2 tsp chili powder

dry ingredients

3/4 cup rice flour
2 tsp xanthan gum

directions

1. In a food processor, chop the ingredients but don't make too smooth. You'll want a little bit of finer chunks for texture.
2. Mix the dry ingredients in a separate bowl.
3. Combine the wet with the dry, and hand mix well.
4. Divide into 4 portions for large sausages.
5. Wrap like tootsie rolls with both parchment paper and foil. Tighten up the ends as tight as possible.
6. Steam for 25 minutes.
7. Completely chill in fridge.
8. Unwrap and reheat. Great on the grill.

Watch the recipe here

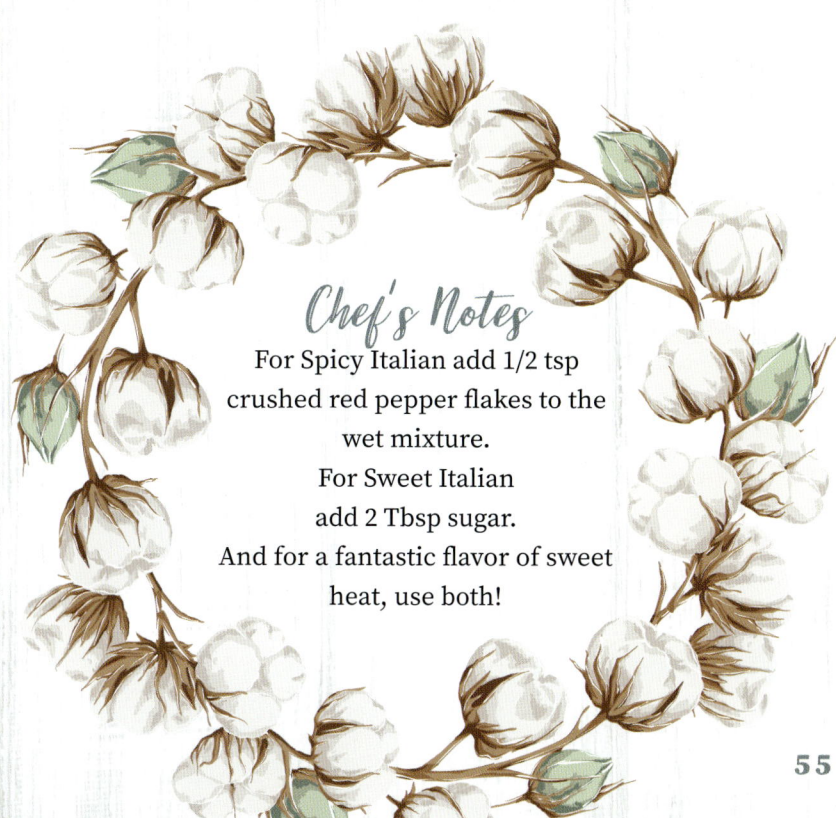

Chef's Notes

For Spicy Italian add 1/2 tsp crushed red pepper flakes to the wet mixture.
For Sweet Italian add 2 Tbsp sugar.
And for a fantastic flavor of sweet heat, use both!

JERKY

JERKY

This is an all time favorite originally shared by Melody Caviness many years ago. Since then, we have developed many modifications to the original recipe. Perhaps you will invent your own variation!

YIELD: 4 TO 6 SERVINGS	PREP TIME: 10 MINUTES	COOKING TIME: 10 MINUTES

THE ORIGINAL VEGAN JERKY RECIPE

ingredients

3/4 cup soy sauce or Braggs Liquid Aminos
1/2 cup water
1/4 cup brown sugar
2 Tbsp olive oil
1 - 8oz pkg Butler Soy Curls

A-1 VEGAN JERKY

ingredients

3/4 cup water
1/2 cup A-1 sauce
1/4 cup soy sauce
1/4 cup brown sugar
2 Tbsp oil
1 - 8oz pk Butler Soy Curls

BBQ VEGAN JERKY

ingredients

3/4 cup water
1/2 cup BBQ sauce
1/4 cup soy sauce
1/4 cup brown sugar
2 Tbsp olive oil
1 - 8oz pack Butler Soy Curls

Watch the recipe here

directions

1. In a large skillet, bring to a boil all the ingredients except the Soy Curls. Stir until brown sugar is dissolved.
2. As soon as the brown sugar is dissolved, stir in the dry Butler Soy Curls, and continue stirring until all the moisture is absorbed by the soy curls. It will become a dry fry situation.
3. Remove from heat and allow to cool completely. Store in air tight baggies.

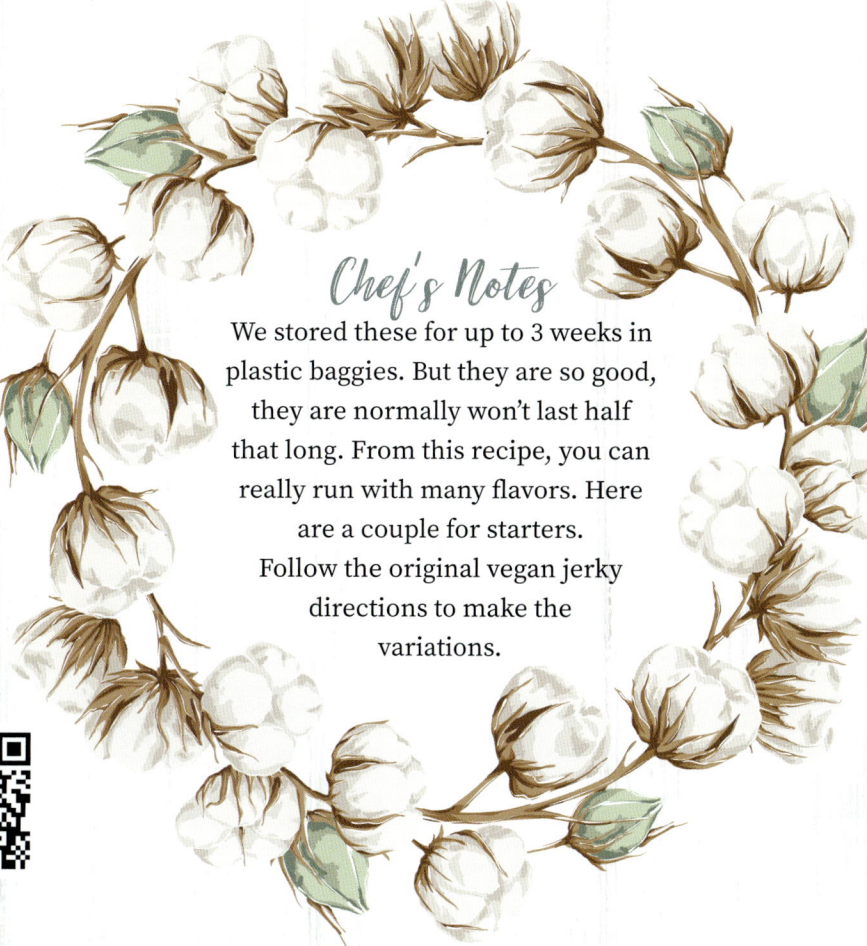

Chef's Notes

We stored these for up to 3 weeks in plastic baggies. But they are so good, they are normally won't last half that long. From this recipe, you can really run with many flavors. Here are a couple for starters.
Follow the original vegan jerky directions to make the variations.

KENTUCKY FRIED CAULIFLOWER

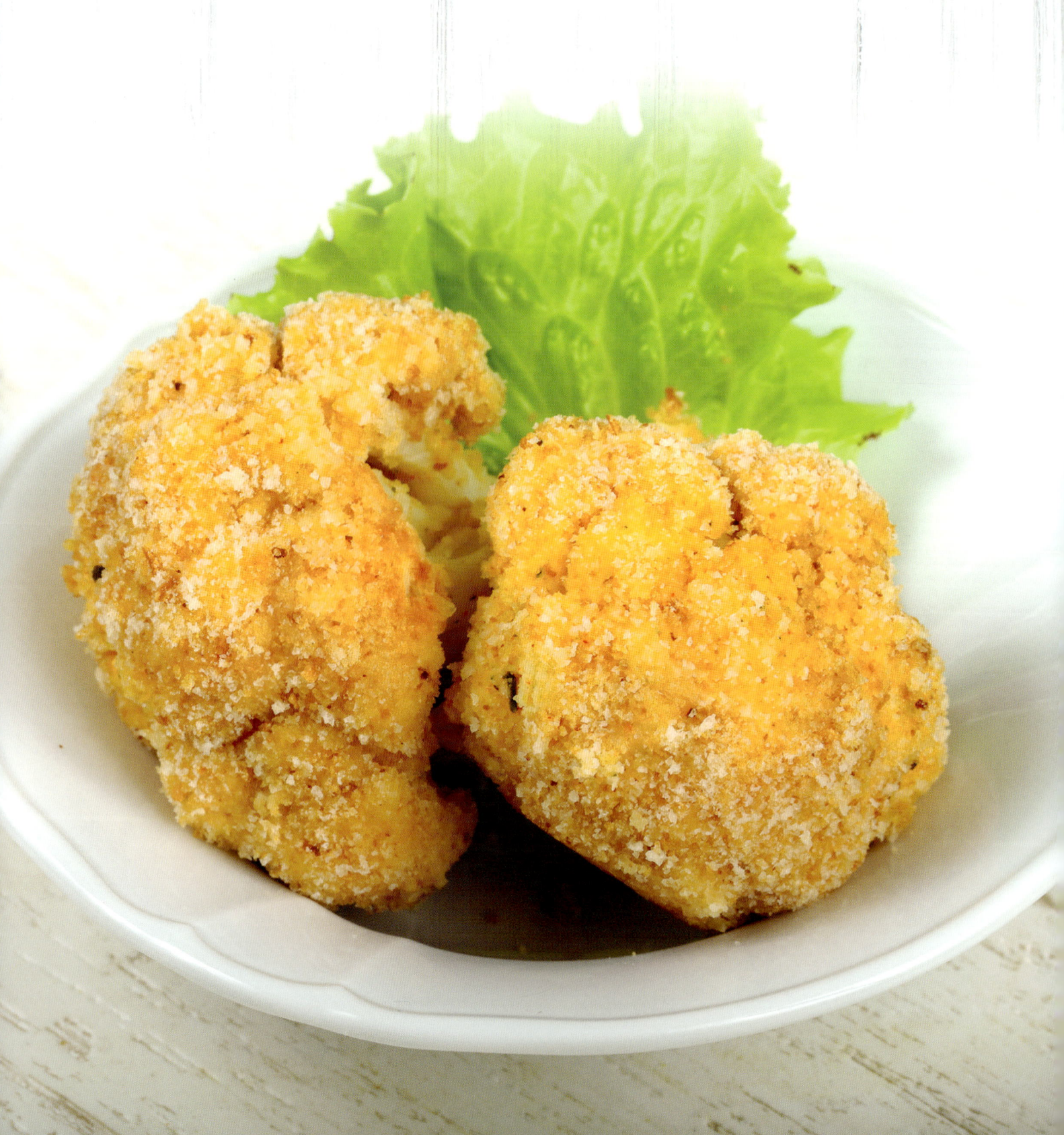

KENTUCKY FRIED CAULIFLOWER

This is it! Chef Mark Anthony's Famous KFC (Kentucky Fried Cauliflower). It's like little chicken wings, without the chicken. Definitely one of the BEST tasting cauliflower recipes you will ever make.

YIELD: 6 TO 8 SERVINGS	PREP TIME: 25 MINUTES	COOKING TIME: 1 HOUR

ingredients

1 or 2 heads cauliflower, cut into bite size pieces

brine mixture

2 cups soy milk

1 Tbsp hot sauce

1 tsp Himalayan salt

buttermilk mixture

Soy milk mixture from above

(See reference in the directions)

1/4 cup corn starch

1 Tbsp apple cider vinegar to create buttermilk

seasoned flour

2 cups unbleached all-purpose flour

4 Tbsp smoked paprika

1 1/2 Tbsp white pepper

1 Tbsp sea salt

1 Tbsp onion powder

1 Tbsp garlic powder

1 Tbsp ginger

1 Tbsp celery salt

1 Tbsp dried mustard

1 tsp dried oregano

1/2 Tbsp thyme

1/2 Tbsp basil

additional ingredients

Vegetable oil for frying

SPICY HOT LOUISIANA DIPPING SAUCE

1 Tbsp cayenne pepper

1 Tbsp brown sugar

1 Tbsp garlic powder

1 tsp smoked paprika

½ cup vegan butter, (Smart Balance)

Watch the recipe here

directions

1. Preheat the oven to 350°F.

2. Cut the cauliflower into bite size pieces. Then place on a parchment lined sheet pan.

3. Bake in oven for 20 minutes, then flip and cook for another 20 minutes. DO NOT OVER COOK.

4. Next make the vegan brine mixture. Marinate the cauliflower in the brine mixture over night, or for at least a few hours. Gently stir a couple of times.

5. Next we will get ready to start frying by first heating your oil to 350°F.

6. Combine all the dry ingredients for the seasoned flour. Set aside.

7. Drain the cauliflower, saving the liquid.

8. Take the saved liquid and add the corn starch and apple cider vinegar, mix well and you have the buttermilk mixture. Place the cauliflower back into this mixture.

9. Now, piece by piece, we are going to take the cauliflower, shake off the excess liquid, mix into the seasoned flour, and then place into the frying oil. I normally try to do batches of 5 to 7 pieces at a time.

10. Fry for about 4 to 5 minutes. If you are going to eat right away, cook crispier, and if you are going to actually finish them off in the oven, you can cook them in the oil much less.

11. When done frying, place on a sheet pan layered with paper towels. If you have deep fried them long enough, they are ready to serve. Or, if you have cooked less, then you can finish off by baking in the oven on a sheet pan (remove paper towels) for another 20 minutes.

12. Serve with the spicy hot dipping sauce. Or a vegan ranch, BBQ, or honey mustard.

Chef's Notes

I highly recommend watching the video on this one. It's the best way to really get all the concepts necessary to make a great product.

KING OYSTER SCALLOPS

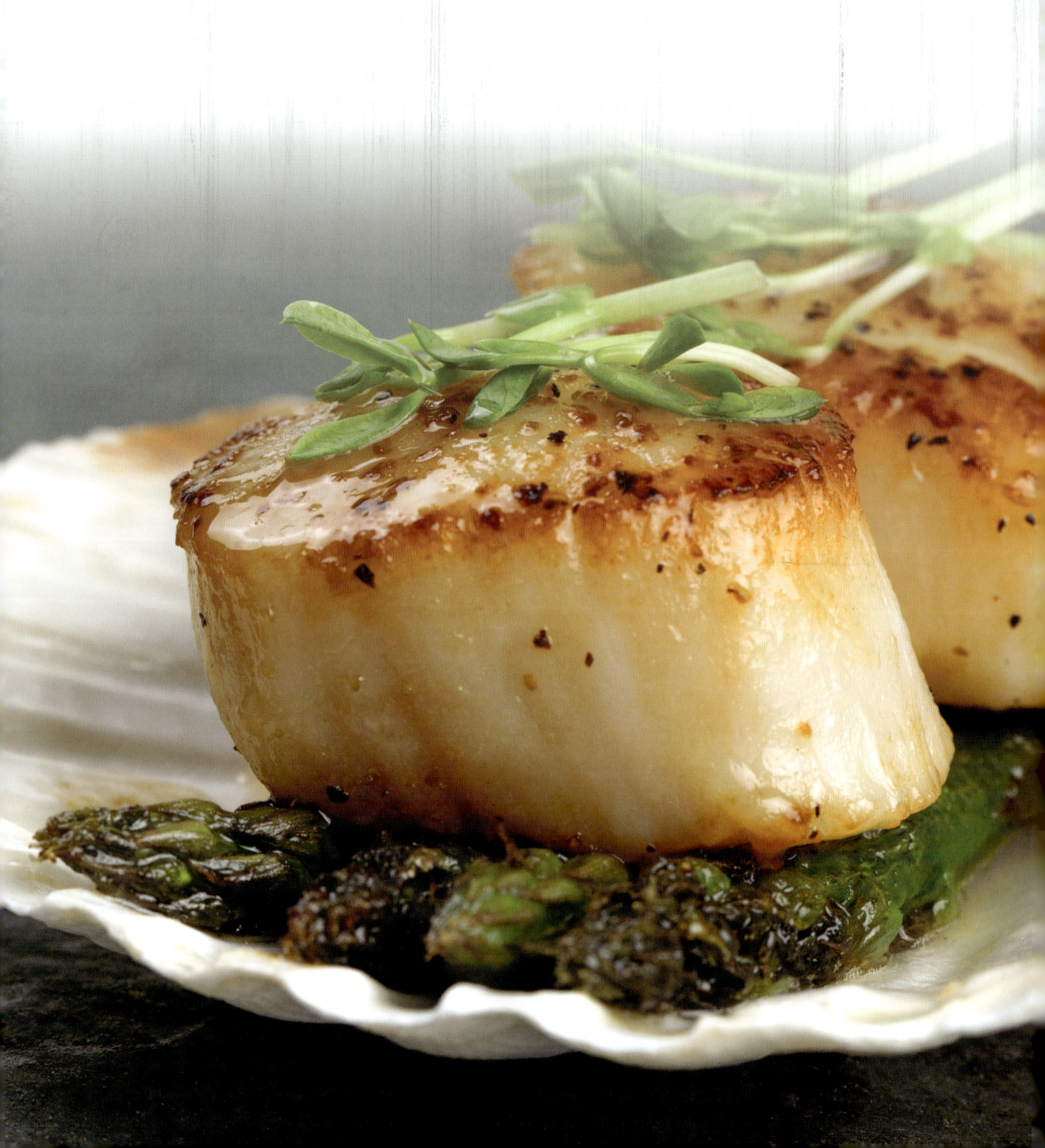

KING OYSTER SCALLOPS

This is a great substitute for scallops. They are so realistic that people really don't know the difference.

YIELD: 6 TO 8 SERVINGS	PREP TIME: 15 MINUTES	COOKING TIME: 1.5 HOURS

ingredients

4 king oyster mushrooms
water
1 cup apple juice
1 Tbsp chicken base
1 Tbsp garlic, chopped
1 tsp salt
1 pack seaweed, or 1-10 inch sheet

additional ingredients

1 Tbsp coconut oil, cold pressed for sautéing
garlic
salt

BREADING & BAKING THE KING OYSTER SCALLOPS

breading station

1/2 cup flour

vegan egg wash

1 cup almond milk
1/4 package tofu, about 1/2 cup
Blend until smooth.

breading mixture

1/2 cup bread crumbs
1/2 cup Panko
2 Tbsp ground seaweed
1 Tbsp Old Bay Seasoning (optional)
salt to taste

directions

1. Try to get consistent size mushrooms. Cut slices 1 1/2 inches each, don't use caps.
2. Prepare a pot of boiling water with just enough to cover mushrooms. Place mushrooms into boiling water and boil for about 10 minutes.
3. Add the remaining ingredients and boil on medium for 45 minutes with the lid on.
4. Allow to cool with the lid on. Or put in the fridge and allow to cool in the juice. This step is very important to absorb the flavors and stay juicy.
5. Pan fry in vegan butter for about 3 minutes on each side, just until golden brown. These are now ready to serve. For an additional method of preparation, follow steps below.

directions

1. Preheat oven to 375°F.
2. For the breading, I will take a couple packs or sheets of dried seaweed and grind it in a coffee grinder.
3. Set up your breading station in separate dishes; starting with the flour, then the soy milk mixture, and then the breading mixture.
4. Carefully bread the cooked mushrooms. Start with the flour, then to the vegan egg wash, then to the bread crumbs.
5. Place on a parchment lined sheet pan.
6. Lightly spray with a little olive oil spray.
7. Bake for 20 minutes, flip and spray again. Bake for another 20 minutes.
8. And Voila - they are ready to serve.

Watch the recipe here

Chef's Notes
Caution, these are extremely realistic.
Serve with a pasta, or salad.

KOREAN TOFU

KOREAN TOFU

This recipe is simply a spin on my old school Korean Chicken recipe.
I've just used baked tofu to give it a chewy texture.

YIELD: 4 SERVINGS	PREP TIME: 15 MINUTES	COOKING TIME: 1 HOUR

ingredients

1 pack tofu, firm or extra firm (I used a 19 oz pack)

sauce ingredients

1/2 cup water
1/2 cup soy sauce
1/2 cup ketchup
1/2 cup raw sugar crystals
1 Tbsp ginger, fresh
1 Tbsp garlic, fresh chopped
1 Tbsp sesame oil
pinch of chili pepper, or chili paste

additional ingredients

Slurry with 1/4 water and 2 Tbsp corn starch
Cooking oil spray

directions

1. Pat dry the tofu to get the moisture out of it.
2. Preheat oven to 400°F.
3. Cut the tofu in any shape you like. My preference is a 3/4 inch cubed, or matchstick.
4. Spray the tofu with a good shot of olive oil spray.
5. Bake for 40 to 50 minutes, 20 minutes on one side then 20 minutes on the other. The tofu should be crispy.
6. Take all the sauce ingredients, bring to a boil then simmer for 20 minutes.
7. Thicken with the corn starch and water slurry. I like it to cling to the tofu.
8. Mix the tofu with the finished sauce, and toss a bit. And it's ready to serve.

Watch the recipe here

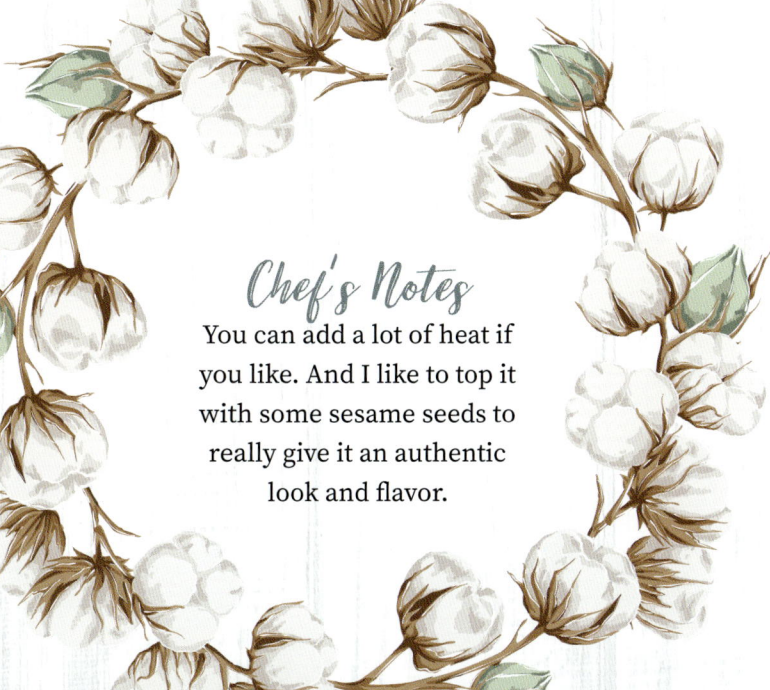

Chef's Notes

You can add a lot of heat if you like. And I like to top it with some sesame seeds to really give it an authentic look and flavor.

MEATBALLS

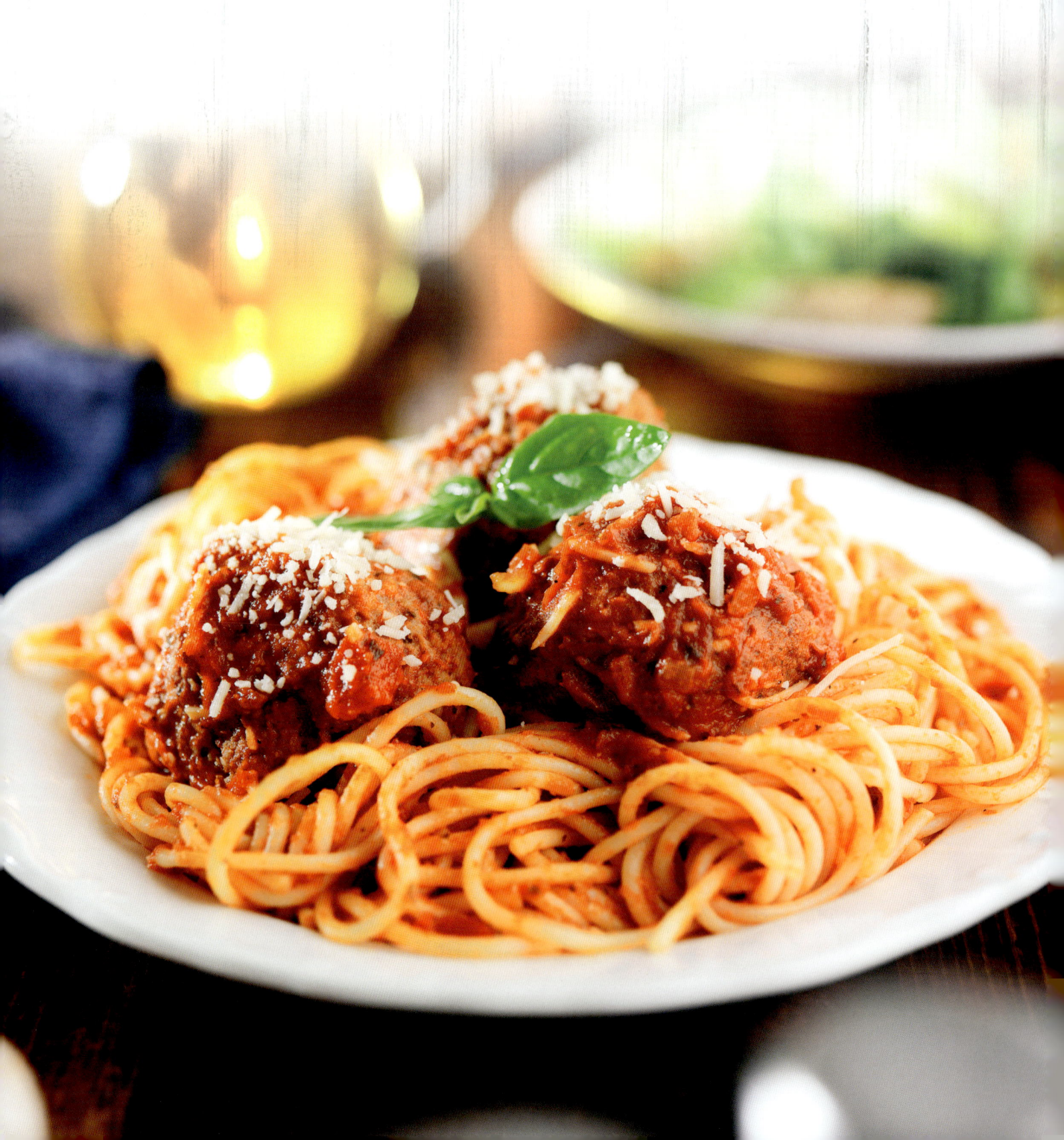

MEATBALLS

These meatballs are a fast and easy version with great flavor and texture. They also hold up very well in sauce.

YIELD: 12 MEATBALLS	PREP TIME: 15 MINUTES	COOKING TIME: 25 MINUTES

dry ingredients

1 cup dry TVP (textured vegetable protein)
1/4 cup nutritional yeast flakes
1/4 cup plain bread crumbs
1/2 cup garbanzo bean flour, or faba bean powder
2 tsp basil
2 tsp onion powder
1 tsp garlic powder
1 tsp oregano
1 tsp thyme
1 tsp beet powder
1 tsp cocoa or carob powder
1/2 tsp smoked paprika
1/2 tsp salt
1/2 tsp fennel
1 Tbsp sugar
1 Tbsp methylcellulose or 2 Tbsp tapioca starch

wet ingredients

1 1/4 cups warm water
2 Tbsp soy sauce
1/2 tsp liquid smoke
1/4 cup olive oil (optional)

Watch the recipe here

directions

1. Preheat oven to 350°F.
2. Mix the dry ingredients.
3. In a separate bowl, mix the wet together.
4. Combine the dry and wet, blend well and let rest for 10 minutes.
5. Form meatballs and place onto a parchment lined sheet pan. Using a #30 scooper you will get 12 meatballs.
6. Bake for 25 minutes. And they're ready to serve.

Chef's Notes

You can omit the olive oil for an oil free version. I normally do a double batch and freeze some.

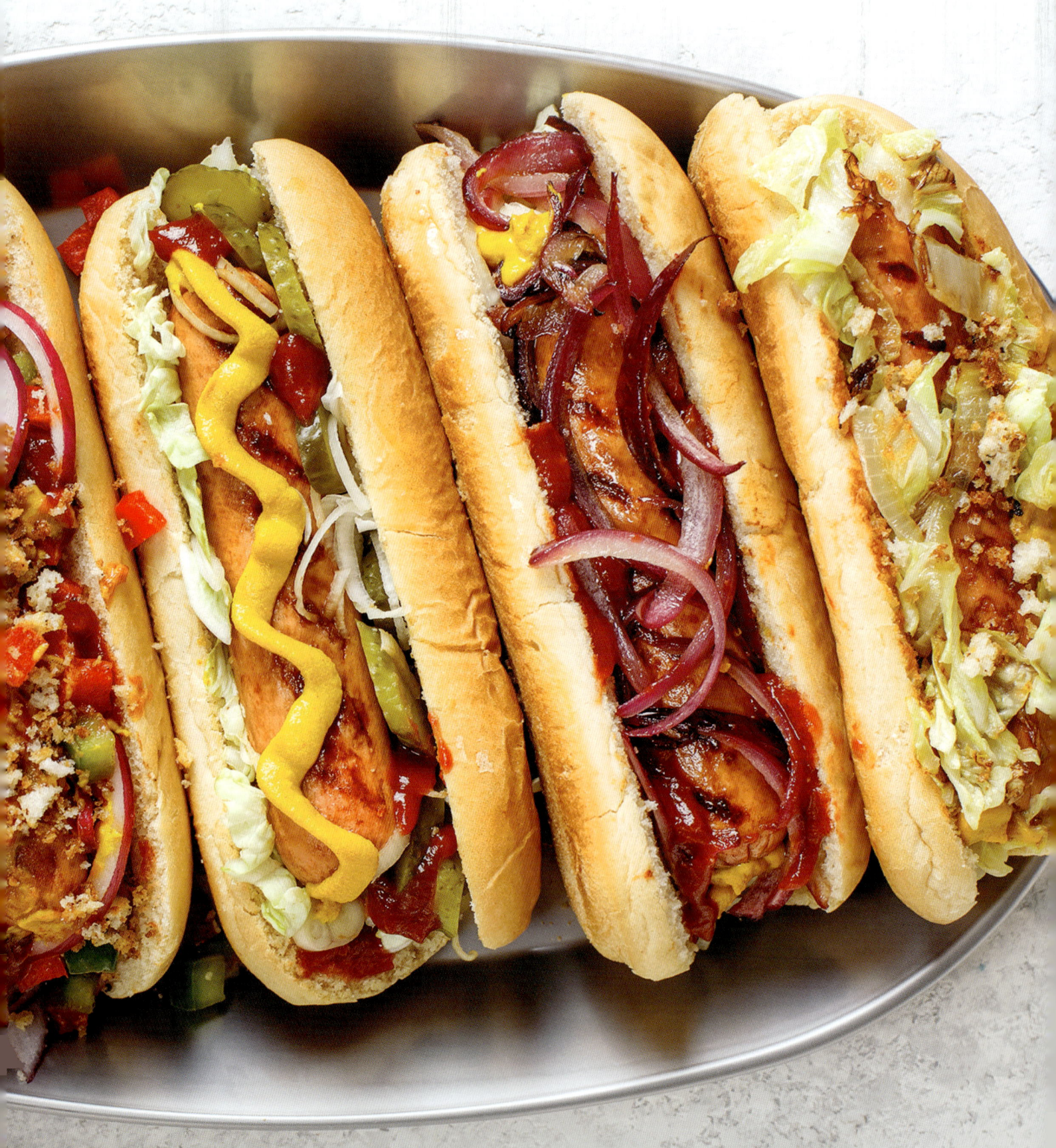

MELODY'S CARROT DOGS

MELODY'S CARROT DOGS

This is a recipe shared by Melody Caviness that will simply amaze you when you taste it!

YIELD: 6 TO 8 SERVINGS	PREP TIME: 10 MINUTES	COOKING TIME: 10 MINUTES

ingredients

6 to 8 carrots, similar sizes
1/2 cup Braggs Liquid Aminos or soy sauce
1 cup water
1 Tbsp liquid smoke
1 Tbsp mustard
1 Tbsp onion powder
1 Tbsp garlic powder
1 Tbsp coriander

directions

1. Peel 6 to 8 carrots into the shape of a hot dog.
2. Combine all ingredients together into a heavy bottom pan.
3. We are going to simmer the hot dogs in the combined ingredients for about 8 to 10 minutes at the very most. We want them to still be firm, but not have any crunch to them.
4. Allow to cool in the marinade. Then place the carrots and the cooking marinade into an airtight container, or a baggie. Let them marinate overnight, or for at least a couple hours.
5. These are now ready to cook. You can grill, charbroil, or use a panini grill to cook them. Get some nice crisp markings on them. And you're ready to serve with your favorite toppings.

Chef's Notes

You can do the standard ketchup, mustard, relish;
or you can kick it up a notch by making a coleslaw or maybe chili dogs. Mmmmmm!

Watch the recipe here

67

OLD FASHION CROCK-POT ROAST

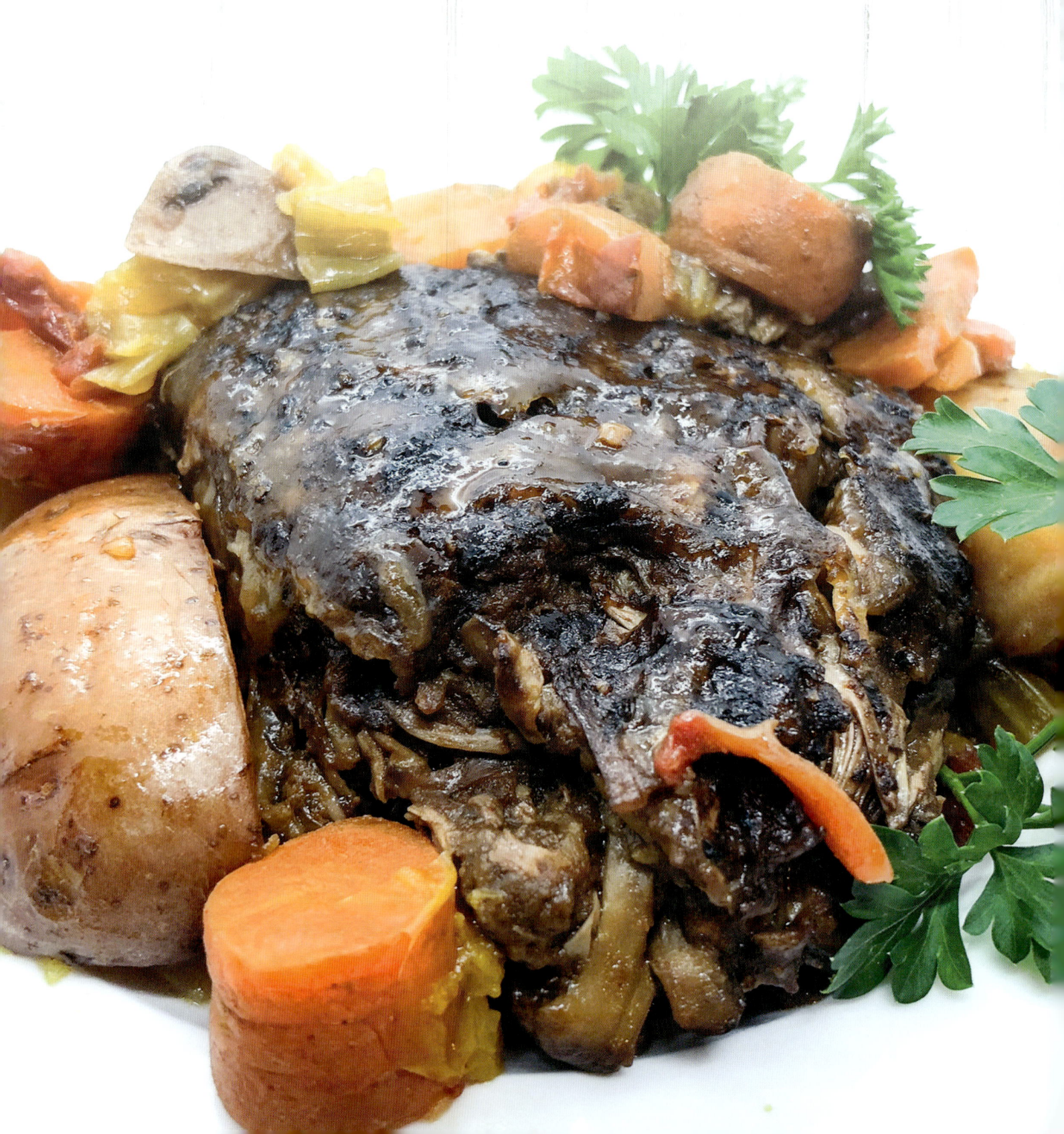

OLD FASHION CROCK-POT ROAST

This recipe is going to fill the home with a wonderful aroma, and the flavors will please the whole family!

| YIELD: 10+ SERVINGS | PREP TIME: 20 MINUTES | COOKING TIME: 4.5 HOURS |

in the crock-pot

4 baby red potatoes, quartered
2 stocks celery, cleaned and chopped
1 large carrot, cleaned and chopped
1/2 large onion, chopped
1/2 red bell pepper, chopped
1/2 - 12 oz can diced tomatoes
1 Tbsp beef-less base
1 Tbsp soy sauce
1/2 cup water

wet ingredients for roast

1 king oyster mushroom
1 can jackfruit in brine
1/4 cup soy sauce
water
The above ingredients will be cooked together.
1/2 - 12oz can diced tomatoes
2 tsp beef-less base
2 tsp soy sauce
1/2 tsp carmel color
1/2 tsp liquid smoke
1 Tbsp onion powder
1/2 Tbsp garlic powder
1/2 Tbsp smoked paprika
1/2 Tbsp chili powder

dry ingredients for roast

2/3 cups Vital wheat gluten flour
2 Tbsp rice flour
2 Tbsp tapioca starch
1 Tbsp xanthan gum

additional ingredients

4 sheets large round rice paper
1/4 cup olive oil

directions

1. Start by boiling off the mushrooms and jackfruit together. Cut the mushrooms in half lengthwise. I make sure the product is covered with water and then add 1/4 cup of soy sauce to the pot. Boil for 30 minutes. When the cooking is done, you will want to drain and cool.
2. Mash up the jackfruit a bit by hand and remove any seeds. Then take the mushrooms and shred with a fork. By doing this length-wise, you will see how the flesh stays in strands. I will then take only 2 or 3 cuts across the strands to make them a little shorter.
3. Fill the crock-pot with all the chopped vegetables, beef-less base, and water. Do NOT add the olive oil yet. Turn the crock pot on high.
4. For the pot roast we will start by mixing the wet mixture ingredients in a blender until smooth.
5. Mix together the dry ingredients.
6. Then add the wet ingredients, the shredded mushrooms, and mashed jackfruit.
7. Divide into 2 equal parts. Each of these portions is going to be wrapped with rice paper. It will take (2) - 10 inch round sheets per portion. Place two sheets on the counter, overlapping just a bit. Soften with water so that they won't crack when you bend them. Then add the mixture in the center. You will want to fold up the paper to enclose the roast.
8. Once the roast is wrapped, sear it in a nonstick frying pan. On high heat, add a little oil, and cook on both sides. This will give it the roasted look as well as sealing up the rice paper to hold the roast together while cooking.
9. Now you can place the roast into the crockpot. I like to put a layer of parchment paper between the vegetables and the roast. Poke some holes in the paper for moisture drainage.
10. Now is when you pour the 1/2 cup of olive oil on top of the roasts.
11. Sprinkle with some steak seasoning.
12. Cook on high for 4 hours. Check on it from time to time and remove any juices that are rising into the meat. You can save this juice and make a delicious gravy.

Chef's Notes

Allow to cool for about 30 minutes to tighten up before serving. Freezes and reheats well.

Watch the recipe here

PEPPERONI GLUTEN FREE

PEPPERONI
GLUTEN FREE

If you're not purposely eating gluten free, that's okay, you can still enjoy a gluten free recipe. Especially something like this pepperoni that tastes so great. I've also made this recipe with about 1/4 of the fat that normal pepperoni has. Enjoy.

YIELD: 8+ SERVINGS	PREP TIME: 15 MINUTES	COOKING TIME: 1.5 HOURS

wet ingredients

1/2 cup water
1/2 cup tomato paste
1/4 cup olive oil
1/4 cup soy sauce
2 Tbsp red wine vinegar
2 Tbsp smoked paprika
1 Tbsp sugar
1 Tbsp fennel seeds
1 Tbsp ground mustard
1 tsp crushed red pepper flakes
1 tsp salt

ADD IN AFTER BLENDING

2 Tbsp garlic, minced
1/2 cup canned mushrooms, minced
1/2 cup jack fruit, minced

dry ingredients

3/4 cup garbanzo flour
1/2 cup oat flour
1/2 cup quick oats
1/4 cup tapioca flour
2 Tbsp onion powder
1 Tbsp garlic powder

Watch the recipe here

directions

1. Preheat oven to 350°F.
2. Blend wet ingredients until smooth.
3. Add the jack fruit, mushrooms, and garlic. Mix well, don't over blend. You want plenty of small pieces in your pepperoni.
4. Combine the dry mixture with the wet ingredients.
5. Divide into two equal portions
6. Then do a tootsie roll wrap with parchment paper first and then foil. Make sure they are very tight.
7. Place into a glass casserole pan and Bake at 350°F for 1.5 hours
8. Refrigerate in foil overnight.
9. Unwrap, and wipe off any excess moisture, then slice and enjoy.

Chef's Notes

If it is a little soft, you can microwave or air fry for a little bit to tighten it up, but I haven't had a single problem with this latest version. For pizza, I recommend dicing the pepperoni into small cuts. That's because there is not enough fat in the recipe and large slices tend to dry up fast and harden on the pizza. For any other applications, you can use this pepperoni like any other. if you want extremely thin slices, you will need to freeze for a while before cutting.

PORK TENDERLOIN WITH HONEY MUSTARD GLAZE

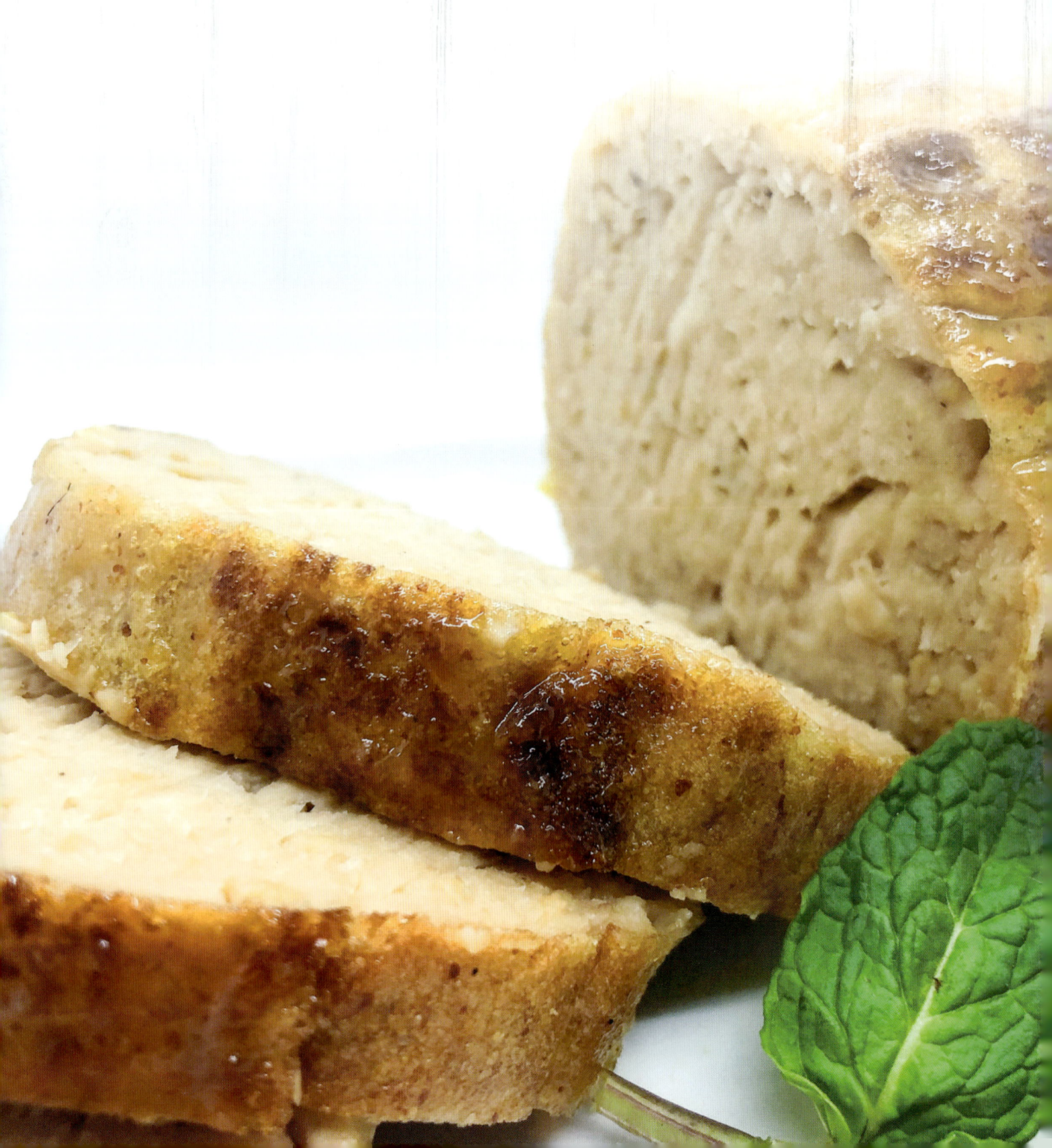

PORK TENDERLOIN
WITH HONEY MUSTARD GLAZE

Don't let the title scare you away from trying this delicious all vegan recipe! Call it a mushroom or bean loaf. Whatever it takes, try it! This will soon become an all time favorite.

YIELD: 8 SERVINGS	PREP TIME: 20 MINUTES	COOKING TIME: 1.5 HOURS

wet ingredients

2 King oyster mushrooms (1 raw, 1 will be cooked)
1 can white beans, rinsed and drained
2 Tbsp apple juice
2 Tbsp olive oil
1 Tbsp apple cider vinegar
1 Tbsp mushroom base
1 Tbsp liquid smoke
1 Tbsp brown sugar
1 Tbsp molasses
2 tsp salt

dry ingredients

1 cup rice flour
1 Tbsp xanthan gum
4 large sheets rice paper

honey mustard sauce

2 Tbsp Spicy Dijon Mustard
2 Tbsp Honey

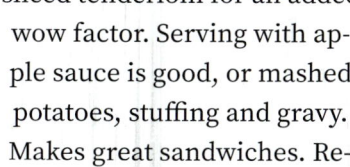

Chef Notes

You can also pan fry the sliced tenderloin for an added wow factor. Serving with apple sauce is good, or mashed potatoes, stuffing and gravy. Makes great sandwiches. Refrigerates and freezes well.

directions

1. Start off by boiling 1 mushroom for about 20 minutes. Cut in into quarters.
2. Add all the wet ingredients into a food processor except the one cooked mushroom, and blend for about 2 minutes, until fairly smooth.
3. Add the remaining cooked mushroom and pulse for about one minute. This will create some texture as you don't want the mixture to be completely smooth.
4. In a large mixing bowl, mix the dry ingredients.
5. Add the wet ingredients and mix well.
6. Wet a cutting board and place 2 of the rice papers overlapping a bit on the water. Sprinkle more water on top so that the rice paper is completely soft and flexible. When softened, wrap the dough. Repeat with the additional 2 sheets of rice paper so that the mixture is double wrapped.
7. Then you are going to wrap first with parchment paper and then foil, just like a huge tootsie roll, tightening the sides as much as possible.
8. Steam the tenderloin in a steamer for 45 minutes. If you don't have a steamer, you can bake in the oven in a steam bath for an hour.
9. Allow to cool a bit. I generally put it in the freezer for 30 minutes. And then unwrap.
10. Preheat the oven to 350°F.
11. Take the roast and pan fry it on all sides to give it some nice color markings.
12. Place the roast on a parchment covered sheet pan and brush with your honey mustard spread.
13. Bake for 20 minutes, and let cool for a few minutes. Slice in 1/2 inch thick slices to serve.

Watch the recipe here

PORTABELLO BACON

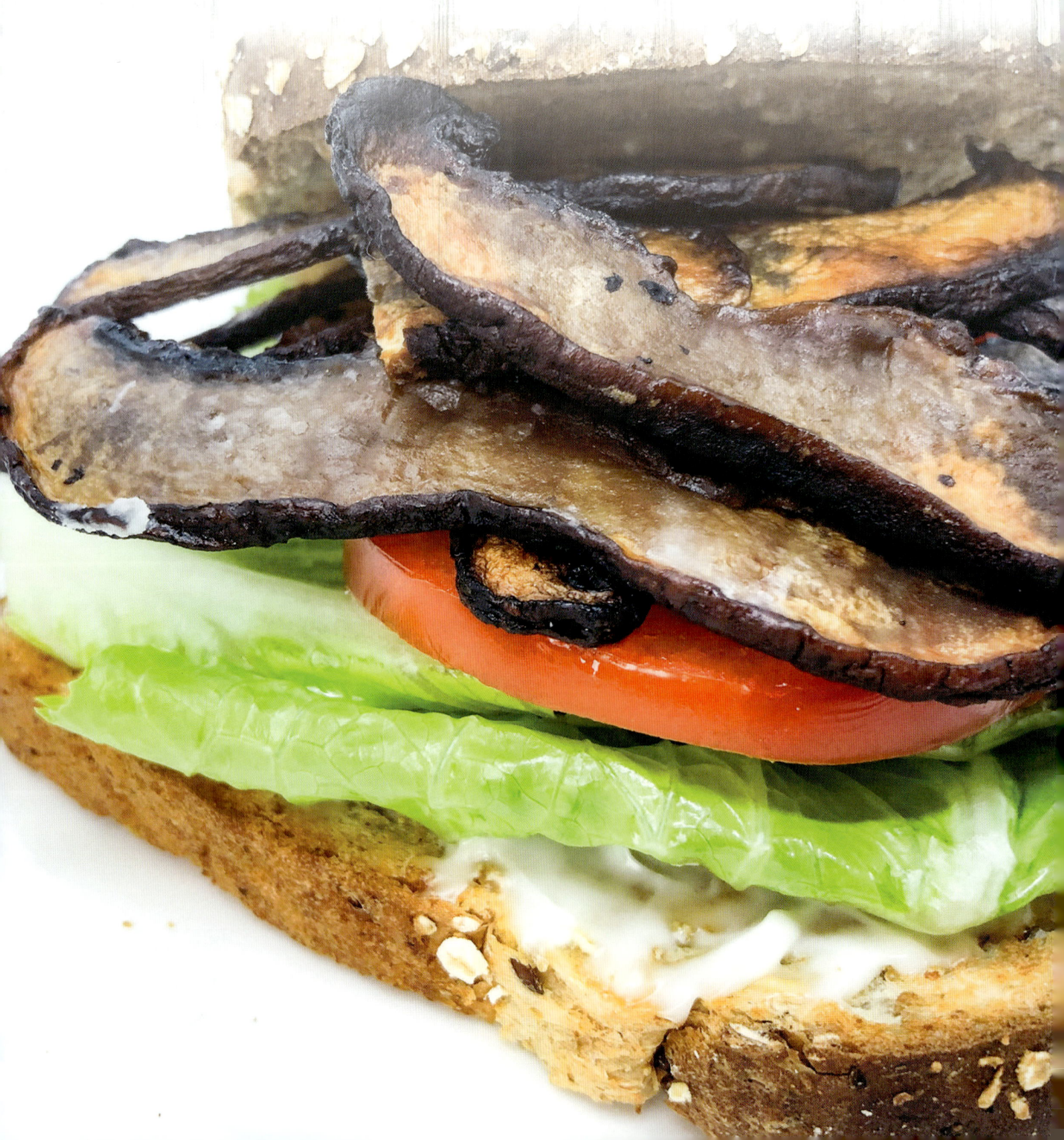

PORTABELLO BACON

For bacon lovers, this recipe will give you something to wake up for. I like to do this bacon as a thicker cut to get more "meat", less fat and double smoke.

| YIELD: 2 TO 4 SERVINGS | PREP TIME: 5 MINUTES | COOKING TIME: 45 MINUTES |

ingredients

1 large portobello mushroom
1/4 cup maple syrup
1 Tbsp coconut oil
1 tsp liquid smoke
1 tsp salt

directions

1. Slice the mushrooms about 1/4 inch thick or thinner
2. Create a marinade with the remaining ingredients. place all into a baggie and allow to marinate overnight or at least for a couple hours, agitate the bag a few times.
3. Bake at 375°F for about 40 minutes or until crisp. Flipping over half way through the process.
4. Allow to dry/cool on paper towels to absorb moisture.

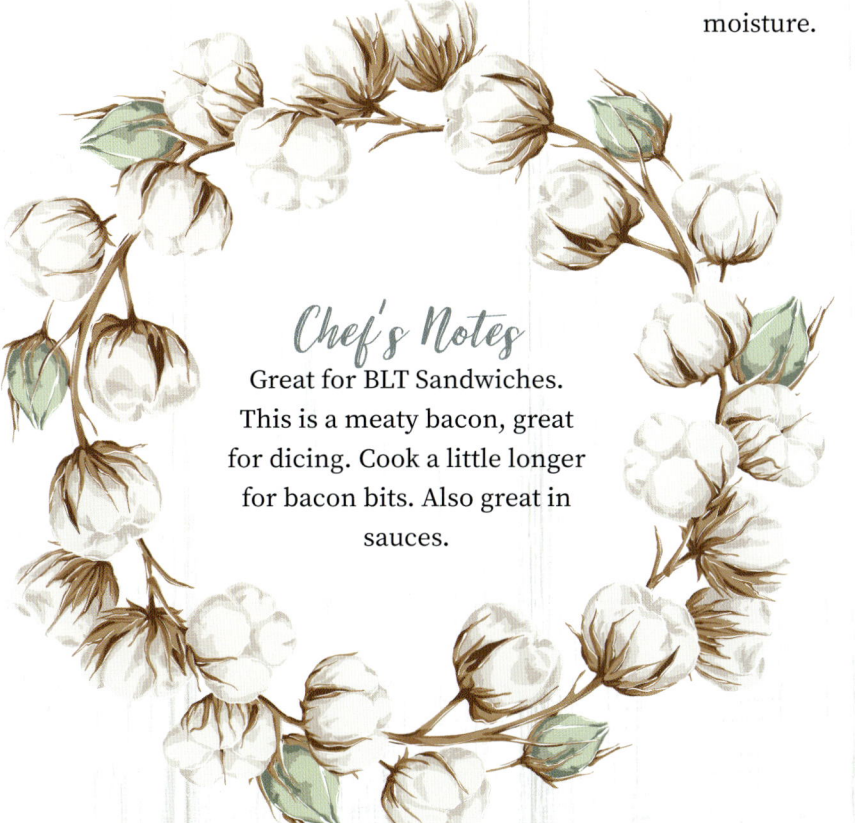

Chef's Notes
Great for BLT Sandwiches. This is a meaty bacon, great for dicing. Cook a little longer for bacon bits. Also great in sauces.

Watch the recipe here

SEAFOOD SALAD

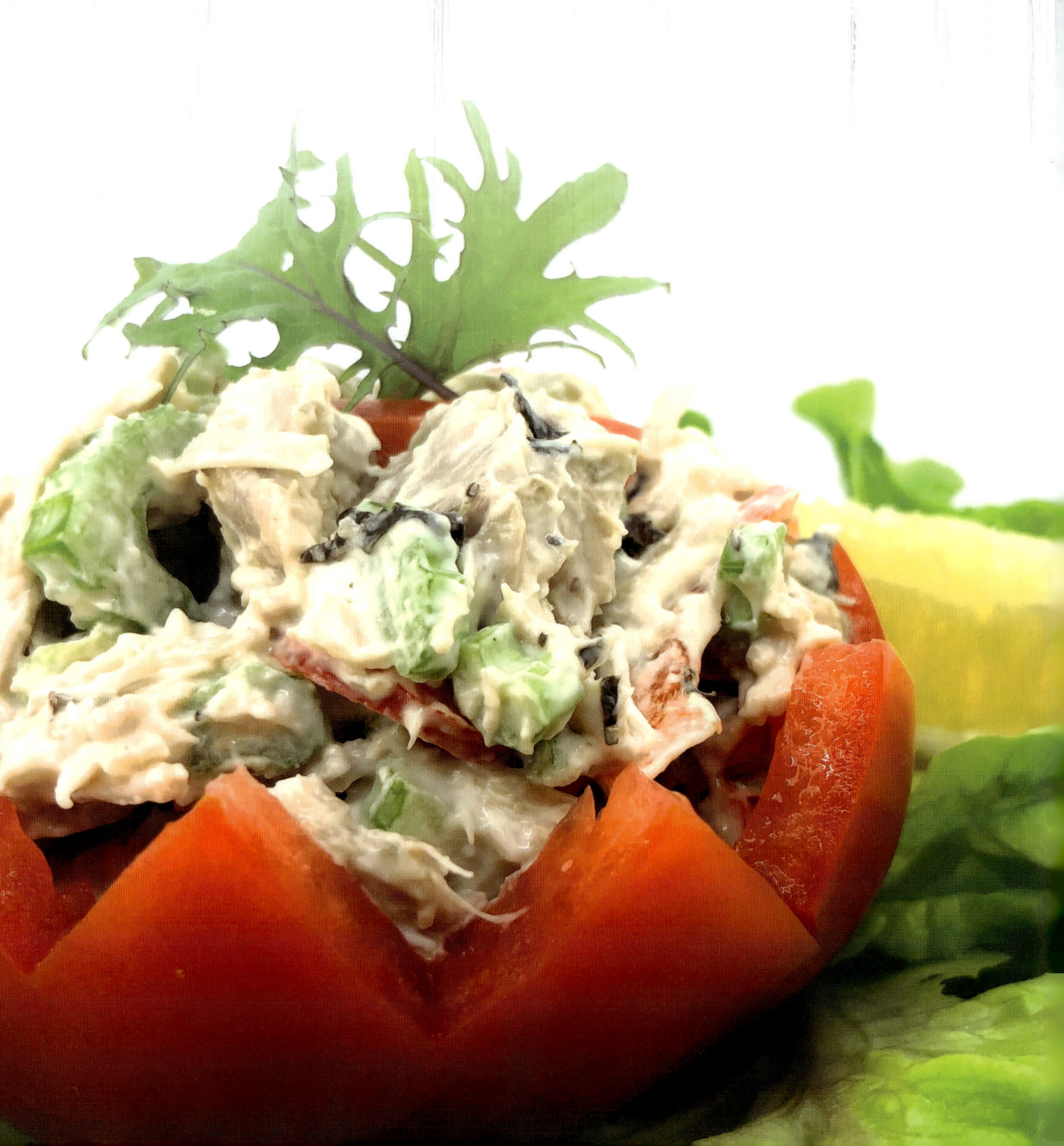

SEAFOOD SALAD

People who enjoy seafood salad are going to LOVE this vegan version.
You'll want to bookmark this page for frequent use.

YIELD: 6 TO 8 SERVINGS	PREP TIME: 15 MINUTES	COOKING TIME: 30 MINUTES

ingredients

2 cans jack fruit
2 Tbsp ground seaweed
3/4 cup diced celery
3/4 cup diced red onion
3/4 cup diced red bell pepper
1/2 to 1 cup vegan mayo
1 Tbsp ground seaweed
salt to taste

directions

1. Remove any seeds or pods from the jack fruit.
2. Place jack fruit in cooking pot, and cover with just enough water for boiling.
3. Add the seaweed and boil for 30 minutes.
4. Allow to cool or refrigerate overnight.
5. Squeeze out as much liquid from the jack fruit as possible.
6. Tear apart to get a good shredded look.
7. Add the remaining ingredients and mix well. I start with a light amount of vegan mayo and add more to reach desired consistency.
8. Chill for a while to let the flavors melt, then remix again before serving.

Chef's Notes

The nice part about this recipe is that it's kind of like potato salad— you can customize it to your own liking. If some people don't like onions, or peppers, just leave them out.

Watch the recipe here

SOY CURL CUPCAKES AND MEATLOAF WITH MASHED POTATO FROSTING

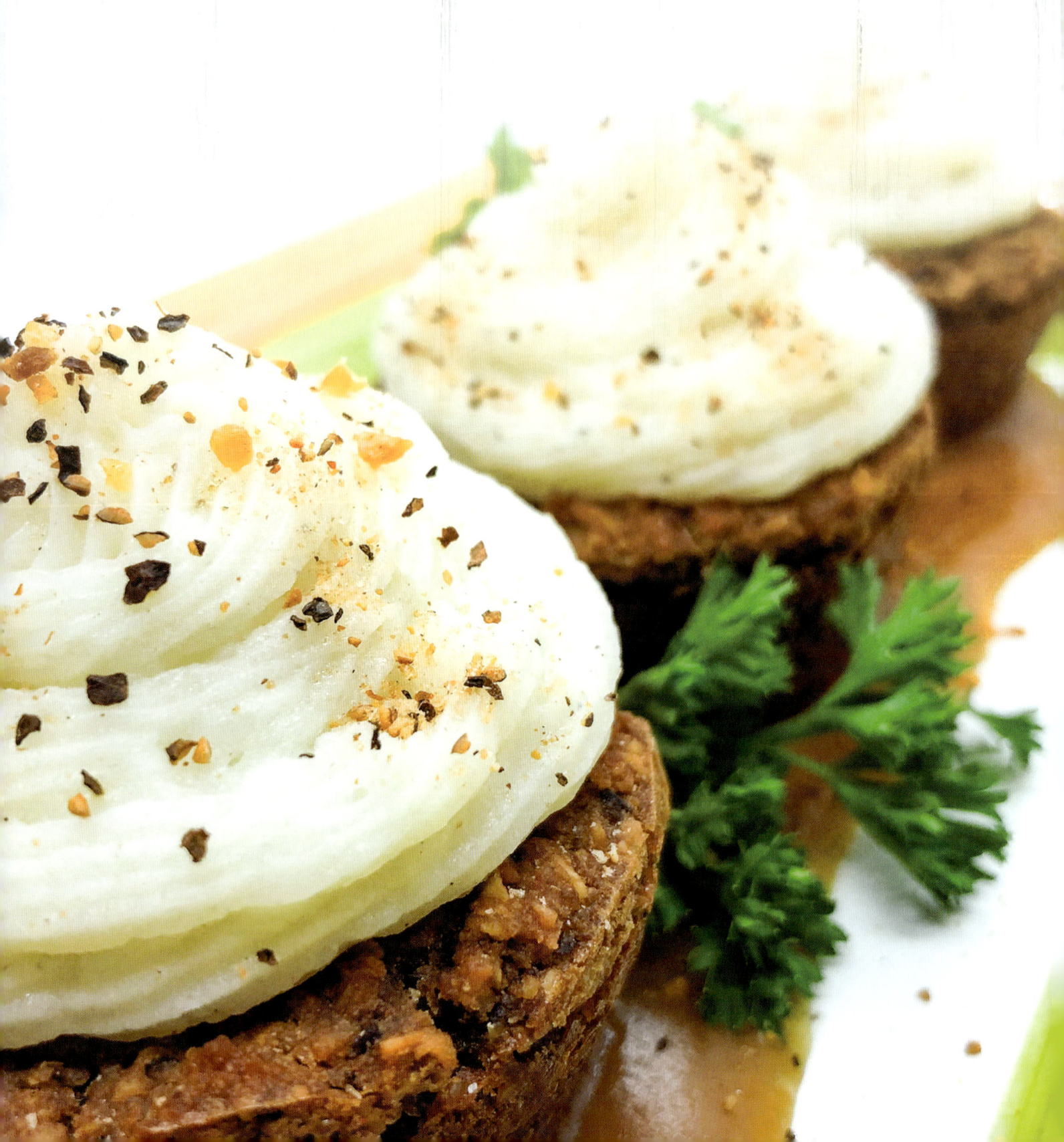

SOY CURL CUPCAKES AND MEATLOAF WITH MASHED POTATO FROSTING

This is a fun recipe to use for either the cupcakes or a standard meatloaf. It is probably one of the best meatloaf recipes I have ever made. Great texture, and holds together well.

YIELD: 9 SERVINGS OF 2 CUPCAKES	PREP TIME: 20 MINUTES	COOKING TIME: 45 MINUTES

dry ingredients

1 - 8oz. package Butler soy curls, crushed
2 cups quick oats
1 cup bread crumbs, plain or seasoned
1/2 cup ground flaxseed
2 Tbsp onion powder
1 Tbsp garlic powder
1 Tbsp smoked paprika
1/4 tsp cocoa powder or carob powder

wet ingredients

4 cups boiling hot water
2 Tbsp Beef-less base
1 - 14oz can refried black beans
1 cup BBQ sauce
1/2 cup olive oil

directions

1. Preheat oven to 350°F.
2. Grind soy curls in food processor. Then place in an extra large bowl with all the other dry ingredients.
3. Mix the wet ingredients together.
4. Combine the wet with the dry, stir well, then allow to rest for 10 minutes.

FOR THE SOY CURL CUPCAKES

In an oil sprayed muffin tin, fill each cup to overflowing. This product will not rise! It should make 18 regular size cupcakes. Bake in the oven at 350°F for 45 minutes, until firm to touch. Allow to cool in the pan for a couple minutes. Then they will be easy to pop out, ready to serve. A mashed potato frosting is a unique way to create an extra special meal. Simply make some very creamy mashed potatoes and using a pastry bag with an extra large tip, pipe the potato mixture on the top of the cupcake to look like very thick frosting. Add your favorite gravy, some sprinkles to the top, and presto, you have a gourmet dish.

FOR THE MEATLOAF

Simply put the mixture into loaf pans. One large pan needs to cook at 350°F for about 75 minutes. Two smaller loaf pans can cook in an hour. Just make sure they are set pretty firm.
You can also splash some bbq sauce or ketchup on the top for the last 15 minutes of cooking.
Allow to cool for a good ten minutes, which will help to release from the pan.

Chef's Notes

To source the Butler Soy Curls:
Link here and buy a big box,
you'll love them
https://www.butlerfoods.com

Watch the recipe here

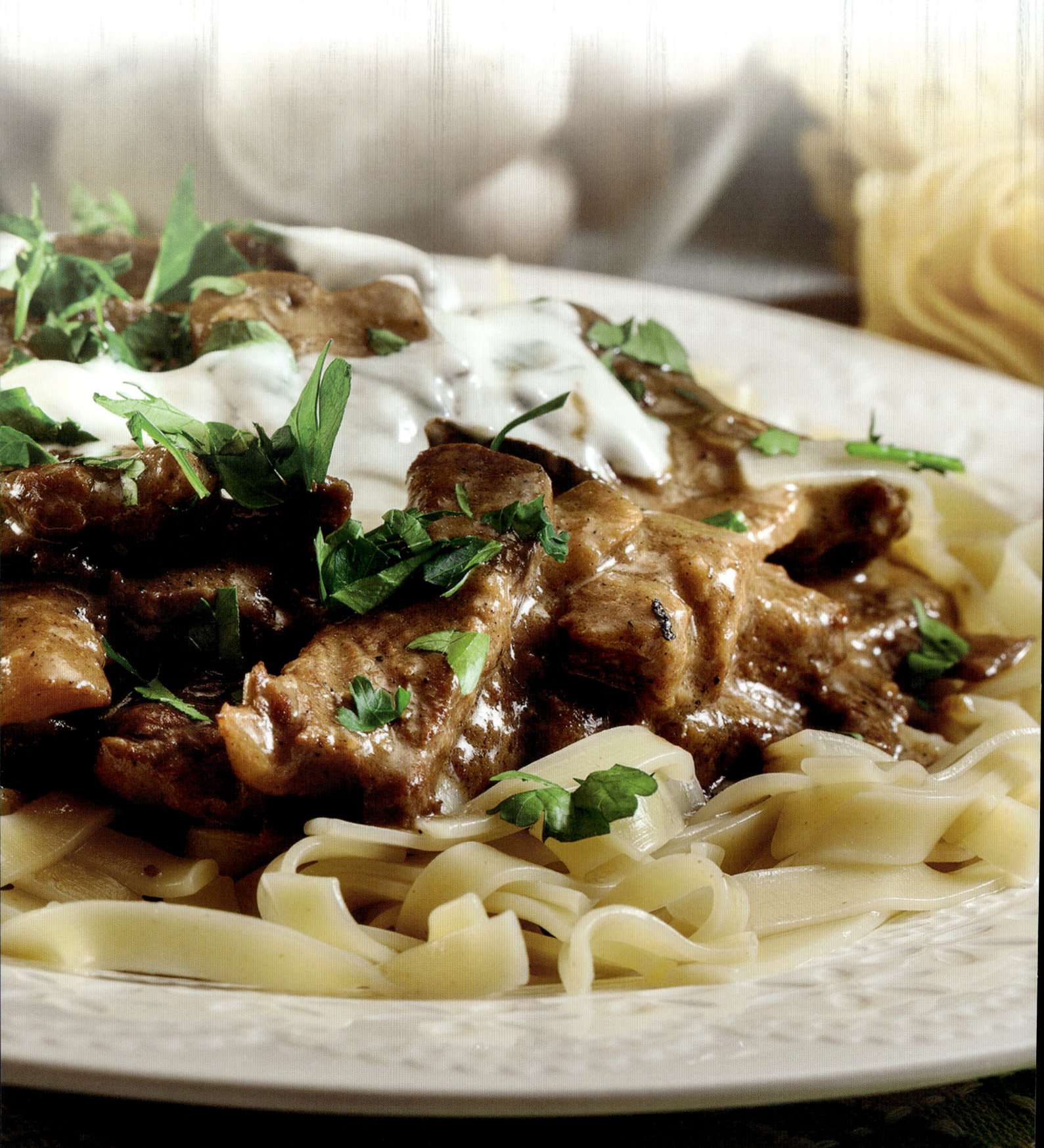

STEAK BAKE FAT FREE

STEAK BAKE
FAT FREE

This is a great recipe to use when making items like Beef stroganoff or Beef tips with noodles.
We have served this as a main course at events with thousands of people.
It's easy to produce, and works well with sauces.

YIELD: 10+ SERVINGS	PREP TIME: 15 MINUTES	COOKING TIME: 1.5 HOURS

dry ingredients

2 cups Vital wheat gluten flour
1/2 cup rice flour

wet ingredients

1/2 cup chopped onions
1/2 cup chopped carrots
1/2 cup chopped celery
2 cups water
2 Tbsp Beef-less base
1 tsp caramel coloring

additional ingredients

1/2 more cup Vital wheat gluten flour
1/2 cup water

Directions

1. Preheat oven to 350°F.
2. Blend the wet ingredients until very fine, no big chunks of vegetables.
3. Combine the wet and dry ingredients, and mix well.
4. In a 2 inch hotel pan or a large casserole pan, form into a log.
5. Poke large holes all over the top and then cover the top with another cup of Vital wheat flour allowing it into the holes. Then splash a cup of water on top of that.
6. Cover with foil, and bake for 1 hour. Then uncover and cook for another 30 minutes to brown the top.
7. Allow to cool, then you are ready to cube for your recipes.

Chef's Notes

This recipe is designed to go with sauces that have flavor. Because it will actually suck up flavor and moisture from the sauces without falling apart, and that's what creates amazing dishes. Great for freezing too. The video shows a double batch. I have adjusted this to make a portion better suited for a family.

Watch the recipe here

SURF & TURF WATERMELON

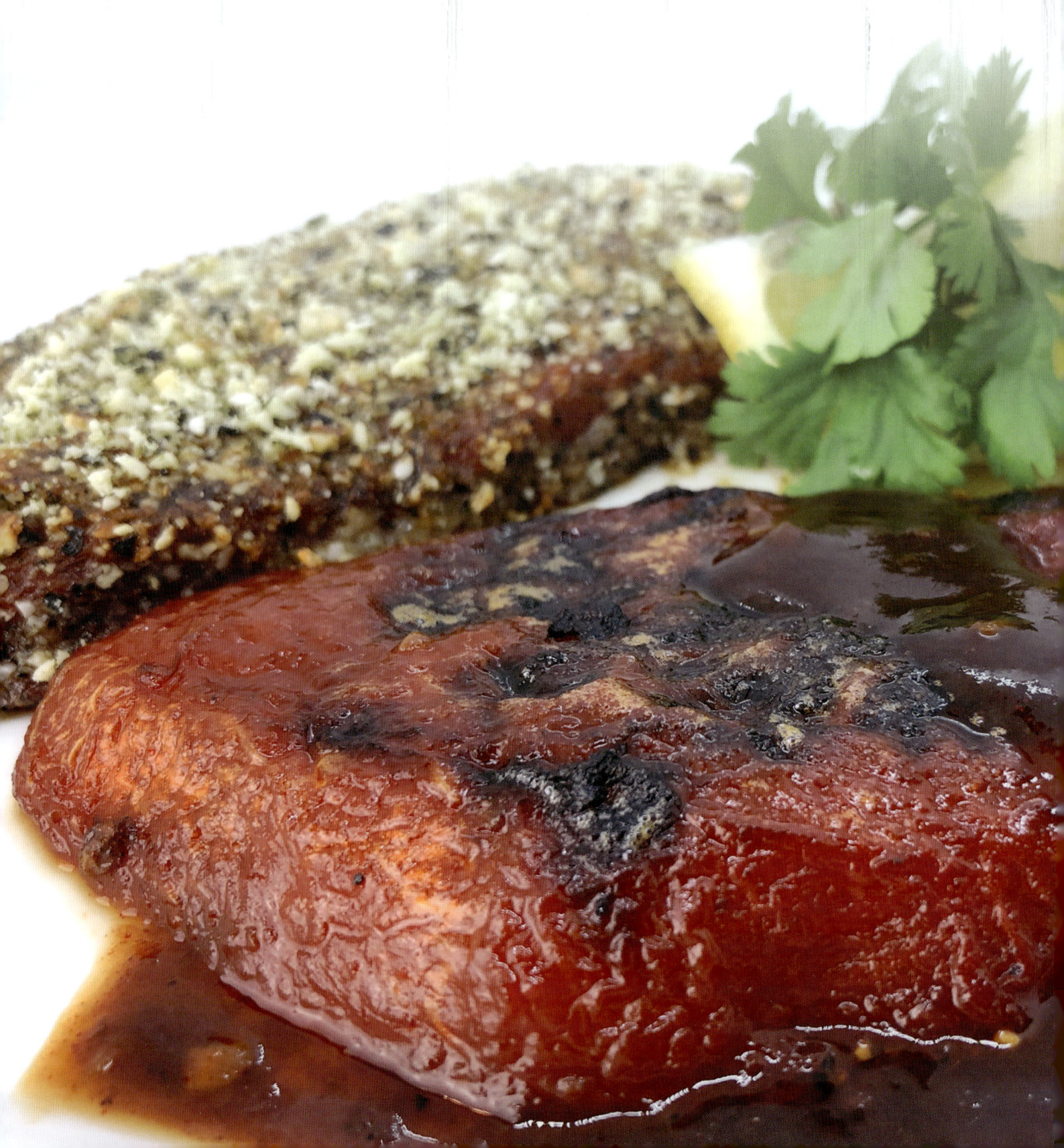

SURF & TURF WATERMELON

If you are looking for a fun and absolutely crazy way to wow your family and friends, this will do it! You can make both variations, one resembling an Ahi Tuna, and another as a flat steak. Both have amazing flavors, largely due to the marinades. And the resemblance to Ahi Tuna or a rare steak are uncanny.

YIELD: 10+ SERVINGS	PREP TIME: 20 MINUTES	COOKING TIME: 3+ HOURS

ingredients

1 smaller size watermelon

STEAK MARINADE
1/4 cup soy sauce
1/4 cup ketchup
1/4 cup A-1 steak sauce
2 Tbsp brown sugar
1 tsp smoked paprika
1/4 tsp liquid smoke

AHI TUNA MARINADE
Juice of one lemon - about 1/4 cup
1 Tbsp Dijon mustard
1 Tbsp honey
1 Tbsp apple cider vinegar
1 Tbsp tahini
1 Tbsp olive oil
1 1/2 Tbsp dulse, or ground seaweed
1 tsp chopped garlic
1/4 tsp salt

BREADING FOR CRUSTED AHI TUNA
1 cup ground almonds
1 Tbsp black sesame seeds
1/4 cup ground seaweed
1/2 tsp salt
Blend together

directions

1. Peel the watermelon, cut in half. and place on a parchment lined sheet pan. Coat with salt on all sides. Bake in a 350°F oven for 90 minutes to 3 hours. This depends on the size, and the water content. You are simply dehydrating it.
2. The marinades are proportioned for a mini watermelon, or 1/2 of a regular small watermelon. If you are going to do more, simply double the marinade.
3. Now this is where you can be creative. First, slice the watermelon to the desired thickness; 2 inches is good and thick. Lay flat on a sheet pan.
4. Stab some holes or slices into the top of the watermelon. Cover with marinade and then bake for another 30 minutes. To finish with an appetizing look, broil in oven, in order to get some chard coloring; or pan fry, or put on the outdoor barbeque.
5. For the Ahi Tuna; drench the slices of marinated melon in the breading. I have tried frying, and broiling this. Both options are delicious. You just need to be very careful, because the breading has difficulty holding to the melon.

Chef's Notes

I like to double the sauce recipe so I have plenty for splashing and dipping. Also, watermelon leftovers do not refrigerate!

Watch the recipe here

TOFU BACON

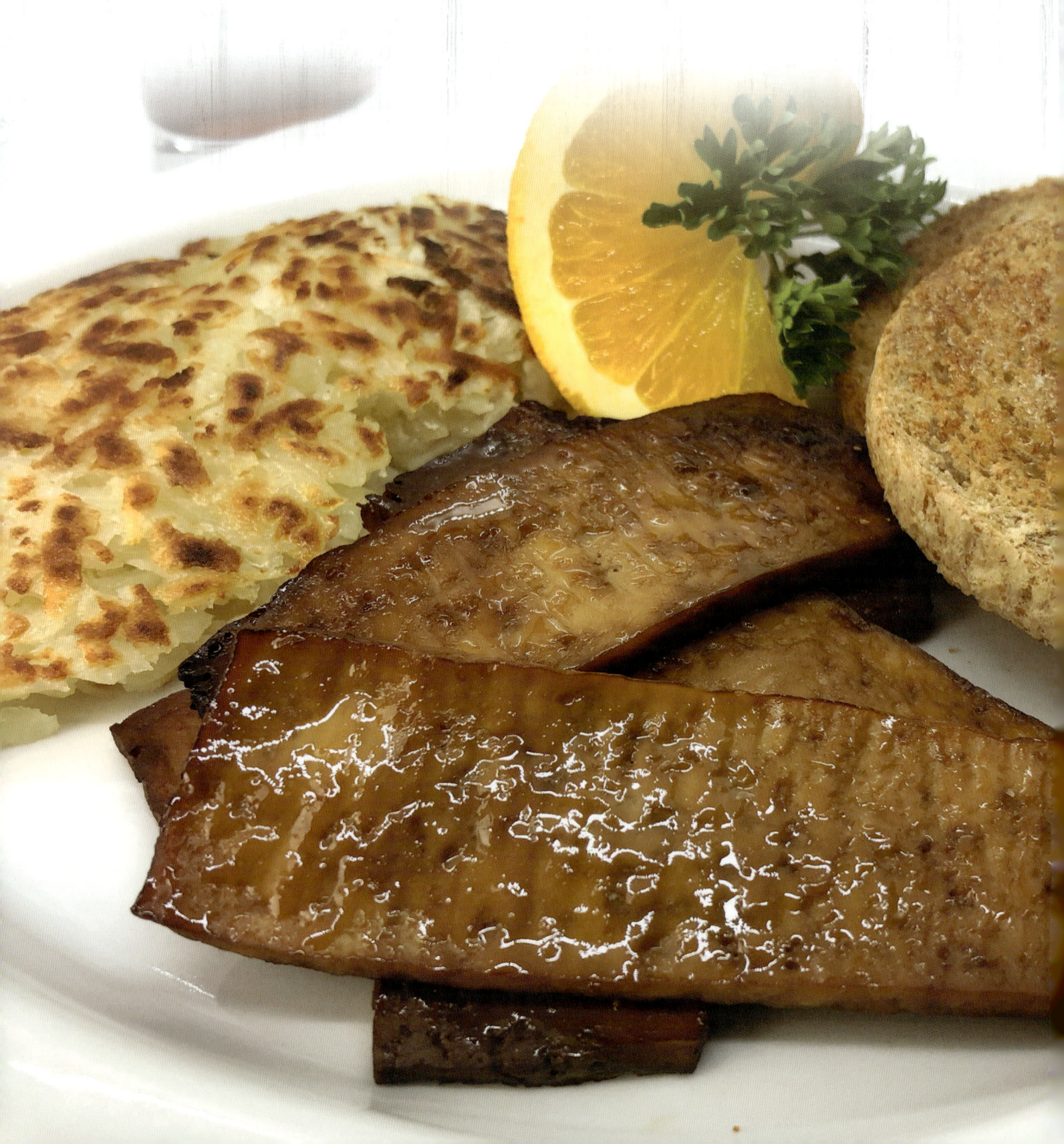

TOFU BACON

This is a recipe that you will use over and over because it is so easy to make, and the flavor is perfect.

YIELD: 8 TO 10 SERVINGS	PREP TIME: 10 MINUTES	COOKING TIME: 30 MINUTES

ingredients

1 pack tofu firm

marinade

1/4 cup soy sauce

3 Tbsp maple syrup

2 Tbsp olive oil

2 tsp liquid smoke

2 Tbsp nutritional yeast flakes

2 tsp onion powder

directions

1. Mix the marinade ingredients well.
2. Slice the tofu into thin slices, about 1/4 or thinner.
3. Lay the sliced tofu on a parchment lined sheet pan.
4. Spread the tofu with the marinade.
5. Let the tofu rest for 30 minutes
6. Preheat the oven to 350° F.
7. Bake for 30 minutes flipping 1/2 way through the cooking process. The tofu should be crispy but still flexible, because it will tighten up as it cools.

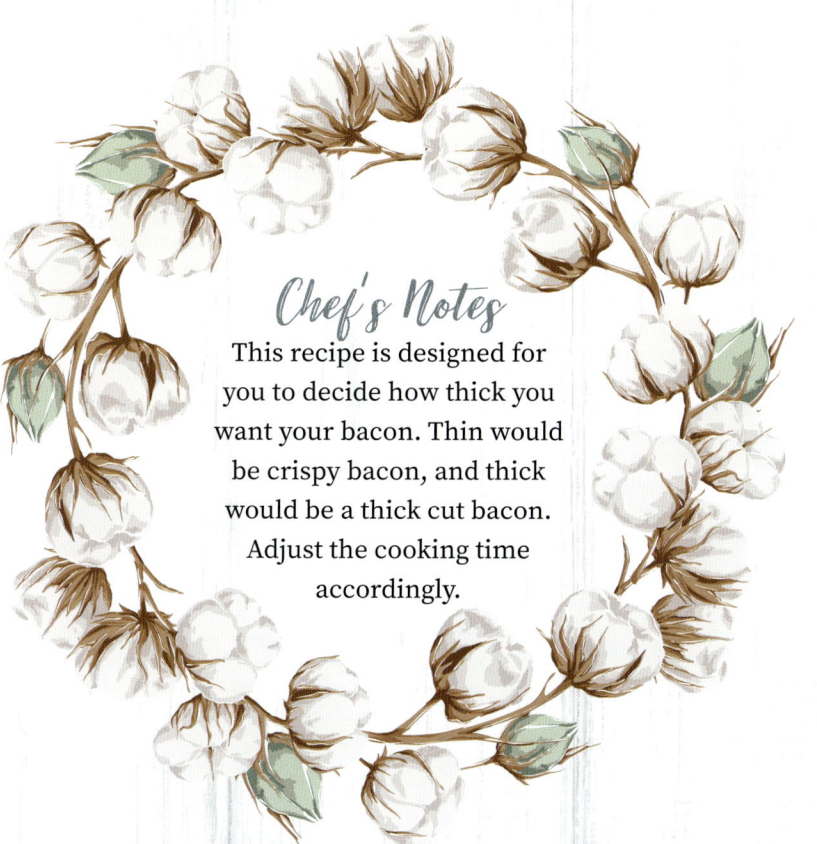

Chef's Notes

This recipe is designed for you to decide how thick you want your bacon. Thin would be crispy bacon, and thick would be a thick cut bacon. Adjust the cooking time accordingly.

Watch the recipe here

TOFU FISH SANDWICHES

TOFU FISH SANDWICHES

You can make fish sandwiches, fish sticks, or fish nuggets with this wonderful recipe.
It all depends on how you cut the tofu.

YIELD: 8 SERVINGS	PREP TIME: 20 MINUTES	COOKING TIME: 45 MINUTES

ingredients

1 package water packed tofu,
firm or extra firm

for the marinade

2 cups hot water
1 tsp salt
1 tsp onion powder
1/2 tsp garlic
2 packs seaweed

breading station

1/2 cup flour

vegan egg wash

1 cup almond milk
1/4 package tofu

breading mixture

1/2 cup bread crumbs
1/2 cup Panko bread crumbs
2 Tbsp ground seaweed
1 Tbsp Old Bay Seasoning (optional)
salt to taste

directions

1. Cut the tofu into your desired shape.
2. Marinate the tofu in the marinade for 2 hours or over night in the refrigerator.
3. Preheat oven to 375°F.
4. For the vegan egg wash, blend some almond milk with tofu.
5. For the breading, I will take a couple packs or sheets of seaweed and grind it in a coffee grinder. Mix this with the bread crumbs and Panko.
6. Set up your breading station; starting with the flour, then the soy milk mixture, and then the breading mixture, each in a separate container.
7. Carefully bread the tofu. Starting with the flour, then into the vegan egg wash, then douse with the bread crumbs.
8. Place on a parchment lined sheet pan.
9. Lightly spray with a little olive oil spray.
10. Bake for 20 minutes, flip and spray again. Then bake for another 20 minutes.
11. Ready to serve with some vegan tartar sauce.

Watch the recipe here

Chef's Notes

These are great, with some homemade tartar sauce. If you have some Old Bay Spice, add a tablespoon to the breading. I don't recommend freezing these. To reheat, microwave if you must, but 10 minutes in an air fryer makes them as fresh as the day they were made.

TUNA SALAD PERFECTION

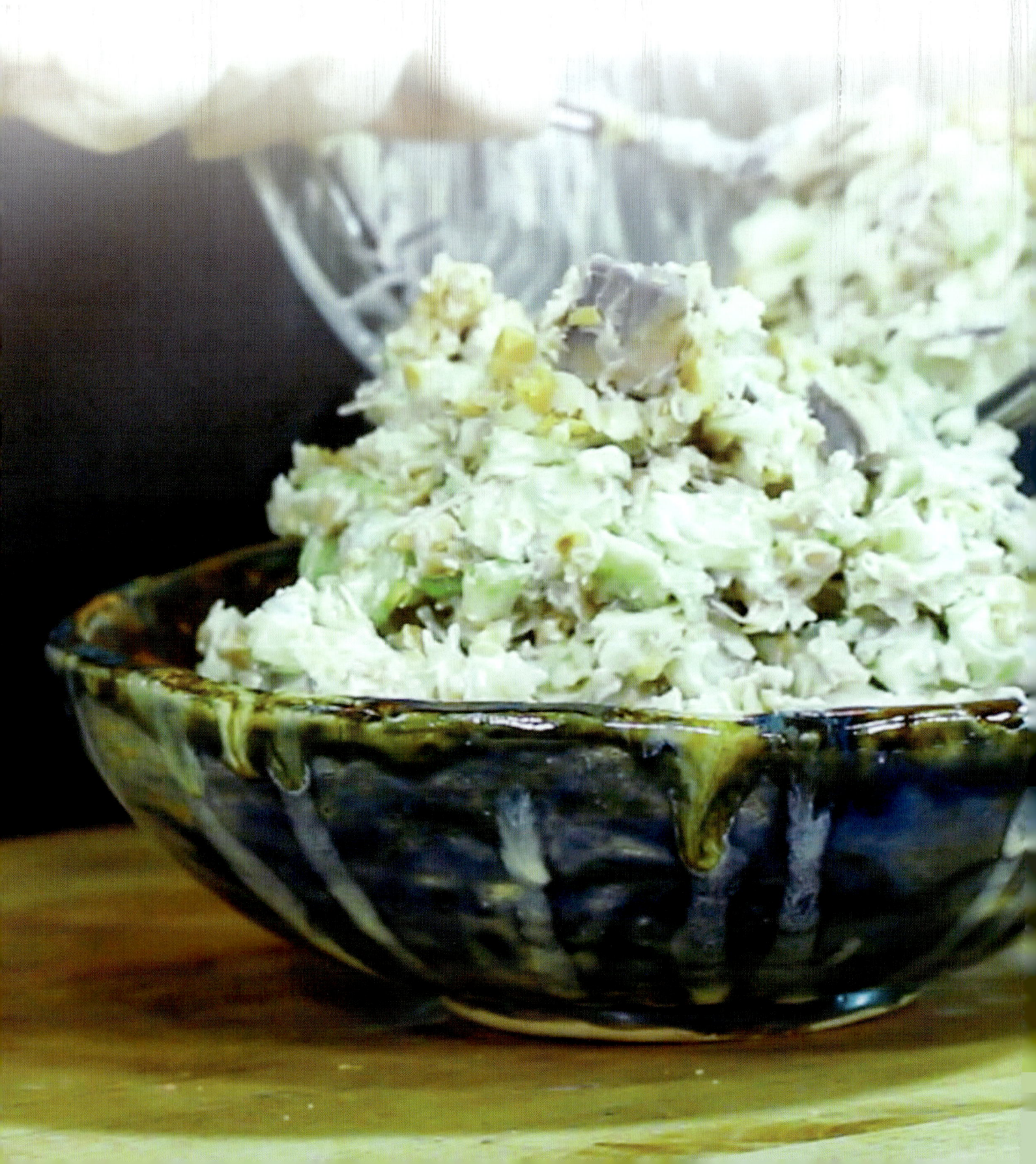

TUNA SALAD PERFECTION

If you're looking for a perfect tuna salad, you just found it. This tuna-less salad has flavor, texture, and is so easy to make. One of my favorites!

YIELD: 4 TO 6 SERVINGS	PREP TIME: 10 MINUTES	COOKING TIME: 30 MINUTES

ingredients

1 can jackfruit
1 can or 1 1/2 cups chick peas, drained
1 cup diced celery
1 cup diced onion
1 cup or more vegan mayo
salt and pepper to taste

directions

1. Boil the jackfruit for 25 minutes and then drain and allow to cool.
2. In a food processor pulse the jackfruit and chickpeas just a little. Don't overdo it.
3. Mix all the ingredients together, adding as much vegan mayo as you like.
4. Allow to chill then remix a little and serve.

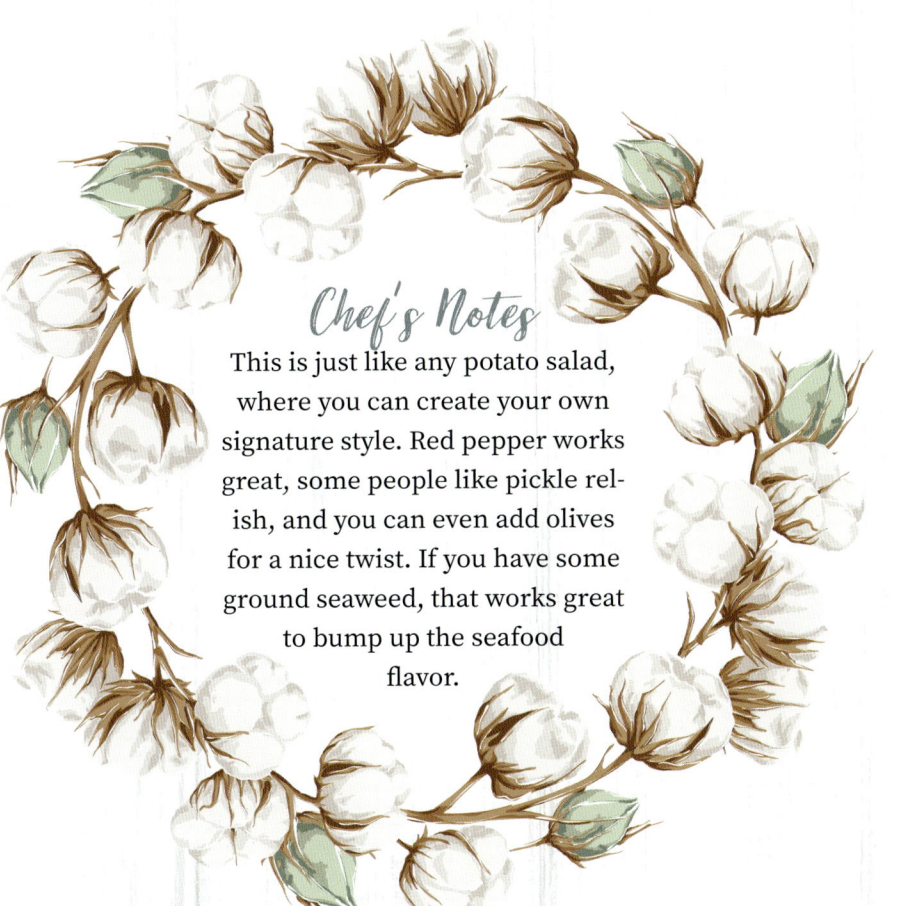

Chef's Notes

This is just like any potato salad, where you can create your own signature style. Red pepper works great, some people like pickle relish, and you can even add olives for a nice twist. If you have some ground seaweed, that works great to bump up the seafood flavor.

Watch the recipe here

TURKEY LOAF

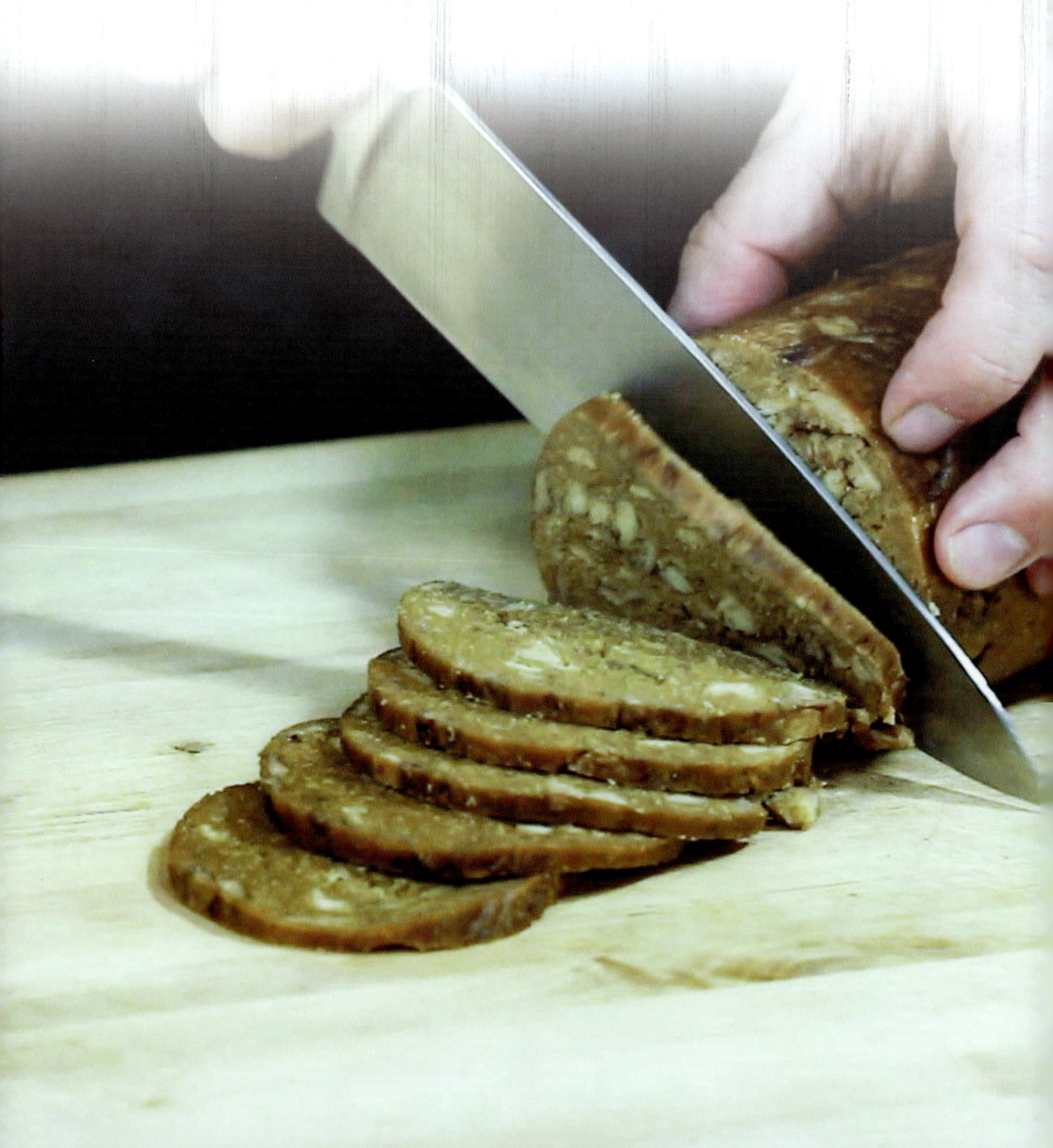

TURKEY LOAF

This is a recipe that started with Melody Caviness. I have tweaked it into a 'chopped and formed' style turkey loaf, thus giving it much more texture. Wonderful as a special entree with potatoes and gravy or a good vegan turkey sandwich.

YIELD: 8+ SERVINGS	PREP TIME: 20 MINUTES	COOKING TIME: 1 HOUR

wet ingredients

2 1/2 cups hot, water
1 pack Butler soy curls (8-oz)
1 1/4 cups oats, quick is best
1/4 cup olive oil
1/4 cup flax meal
2 Tbsp chicken-less base
2 Tbsp beef-less base
1 Tbsp onion powder
1 Tbsp garlic powder
1 Tbsp smoked paprika
1 Tbsp McKays Chicken style seasoning
1 Tbsp poultry seasoning

dry ingredients

1 cup Vital wheat gluten flour
1/4 cup tapioca starch

additional ingredients

1 pack Butler Soy Curls (8-oz), soaked and squeeze drained

directions

1. Preheat oven to 350°F.
2. Take 1 package (8 oz) Butler Soy Curls and soak in hot water.
3. In a food processor, blend all the wet ingredients. Blend for a good 3 minutes.
4. Squeeze the Soy Curls that are soaking to get them as dry as possible.
5. In a large bowl, mix the dry ingredients. Add the wet ingredients along with the soaked and drained Soy Curls. Mix well for a good 3 minutes. Really press this mixture together. This creates some elastic properties and helps hold the loaf together. Form into a log shape.
6. Wrap like a tootsie roll. First in a large sheet of parchment paper, and then twice with large sheets of foil.
7. Bake for 1 hour.
8. Allow to cool 20 - 30 minutes in foil before slicing.

Watch the recipe here

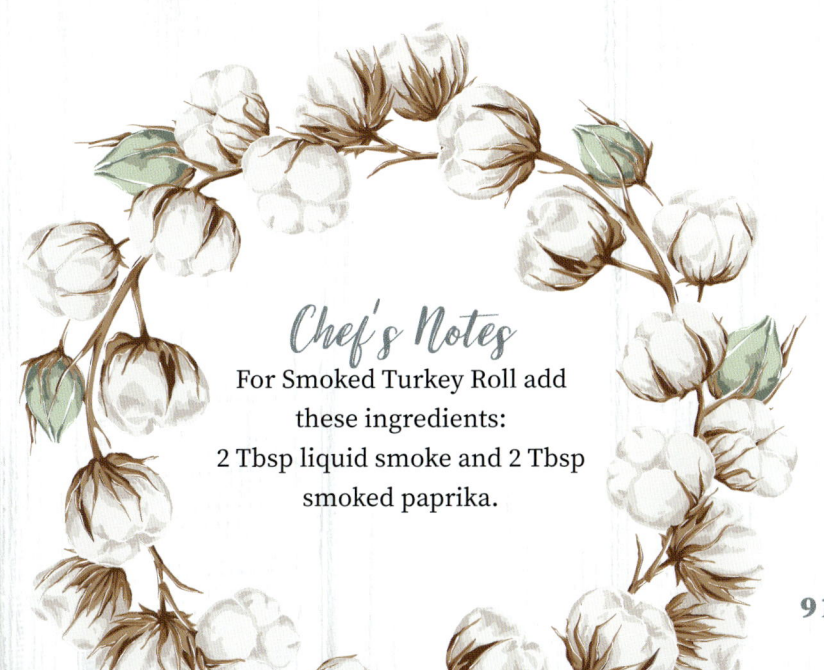

Chef's Notes
For Smoked Turkey Roll add these ingredients:
2 Tbsp liquid smoke and 2 Tbsp smoked paprika.

91

TURKEY SALAD

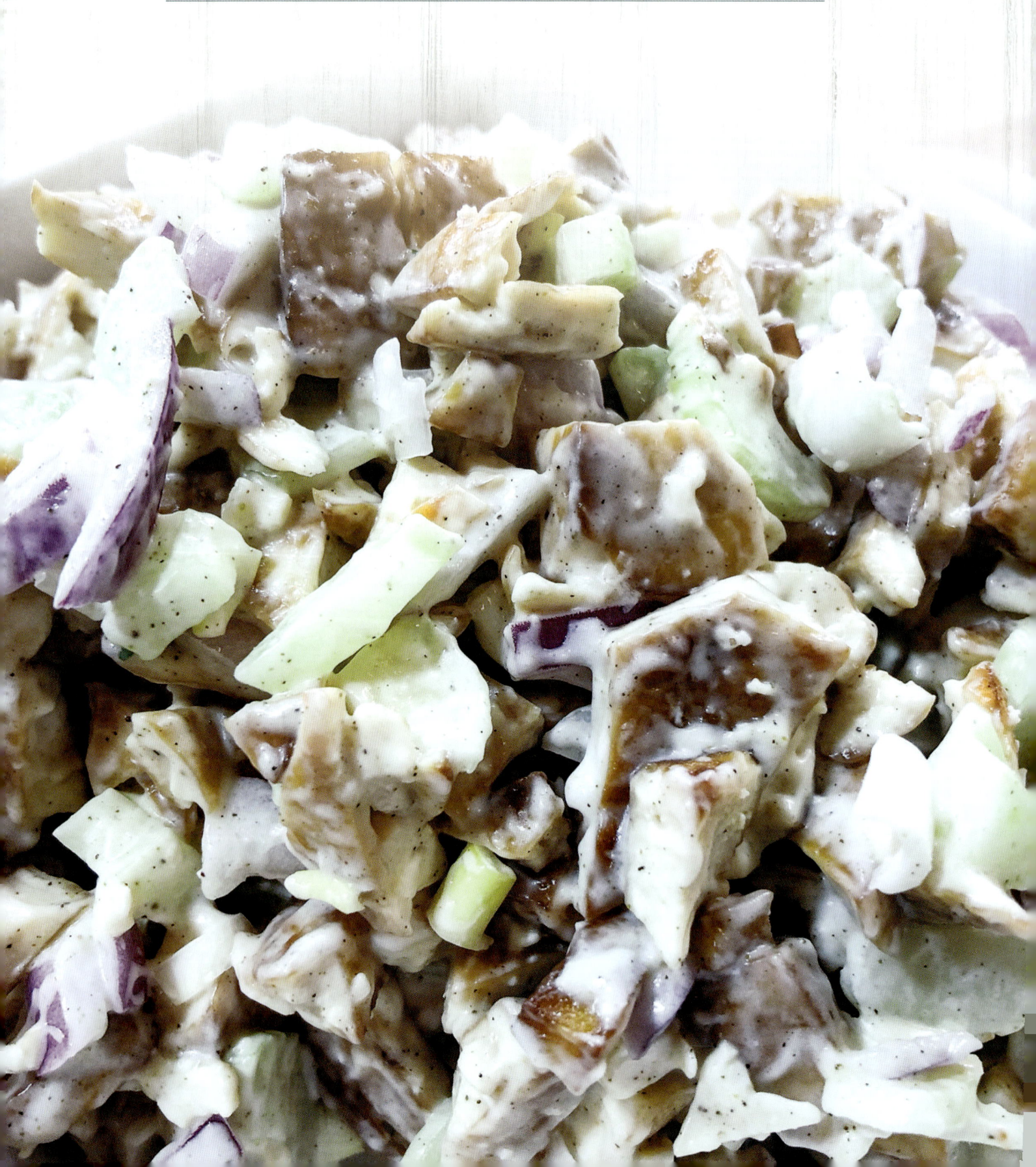

TURKEY SALAD

This is a rather unique way to prepare tofu. A nice variation from the traditional eggless, egg salad.

YIELD: 6 TO 8 SERVINGS	PREP TIME: 15 MINUTES	COOKING TIME: 30 MINUTES

for the turkey ingredients

1 block firm tofu (19oz)
1/2 cup hot water
1 tsp chicken-less base
1 tsp beef-less base
2 Tbsp soy sauce

for the salad ingredients

1/2 cup chopped celery - about one stalk
1/4 cup diced red onions
1 tsp McKay's chicken style seasoning OR
1/2 tsp salt
1/4 tsp poultry seasoning
1/4 tsp sage
1/2 cup vegan mayo

directions

1. Preheat oven to 350°F.
2. Slice tofu into about 1/6 inch slices and lay flat on a parchment lined sheet pan.
3. Mix well the hot water, bases, and soy sauce.
4. Drizzle over the tofu.
5. Bake for about 30 minutes on each side until slightly crispy on the outside yet tender on the inside.
6. Allow to cool and chop into random small pieces.
7. In a mixing bowl, combine all the ingredients.
8. This is ready to serve or chill for later use.

Watch the recipe here

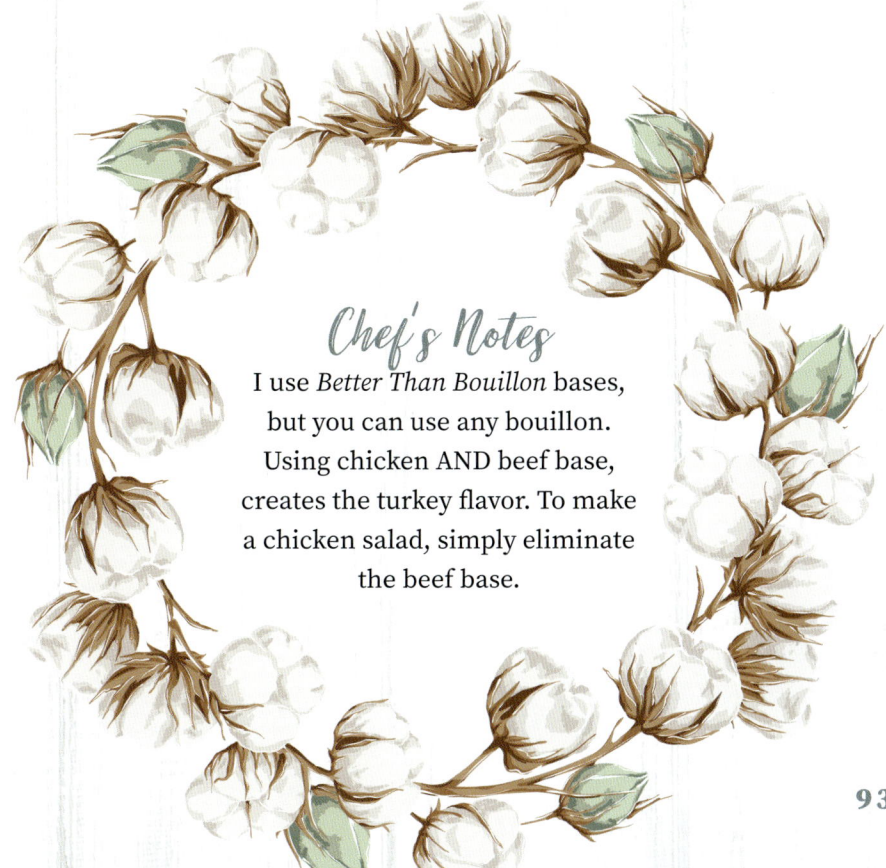

Chef's Notes

I use *Better Than Bouillon* bases, but you can use any bouillon. Using chicken AND beef base, creates the turkey flavor. To make a chicken salad, simply eliminate the beef base.

VEGAN CUTLETS

VEGAN CUTLETS

This is an old time favorite that I've have done hundreds of times at cooking events all over the country. It's easy and tastes great.

YIELD: 4 SERVINGS	PREP TIME: 20 MINUTES	COOKING TIME: 30 MINUTES

for the dough

2 cups water
2 cups Vital wheat gluten flour

boiling ingredients

1/2 gallon water
1/2 cup soy sauce or Bragg's Liquid Aminos
1/4 cup chopped garlic

for the breading

2 cups bread crumbs
olive oil for sautéing

directions

1. Mix the water and gluten flour (must mix quickly in order for it to get the right consistency) and then roll into a log about 2 inches round. Allow to rest for ten minutes.
2. In a medium cooking pan with a cover, bring the boiling ingredients to a boil.
3. Slice the log into 1/2 inch slices, gently manipulating them into a cutlet shape, and drop into the boiling water one at a time. When done, give a light stir. Turn the heat down to medium for a light rolling boil.
4. Boil with the lid on for 20 to 25 minutes, lightly stirring a couple times.
5. Drain, and cool. Then squeeze extra juice out of the cutlets.
6. Now all you have to do is bread the cutlets and pan fry with a little olive oil until crispy golden on both sides. They are ready to serve.

Chef's Notes

These are great to make and serve with a rice or potato dish, or for sandwiches, even dipping like chicken nuggets. I do not recommend freezing, because they tend to get really rubbery and tough. I've done southwest style with southwest seasonings in the breading, or Italian cutlets with a 1/4 cup of Italian seasoning added to the bread crumbs.

Watch the recipe here

VEGAN RIBS 4.0

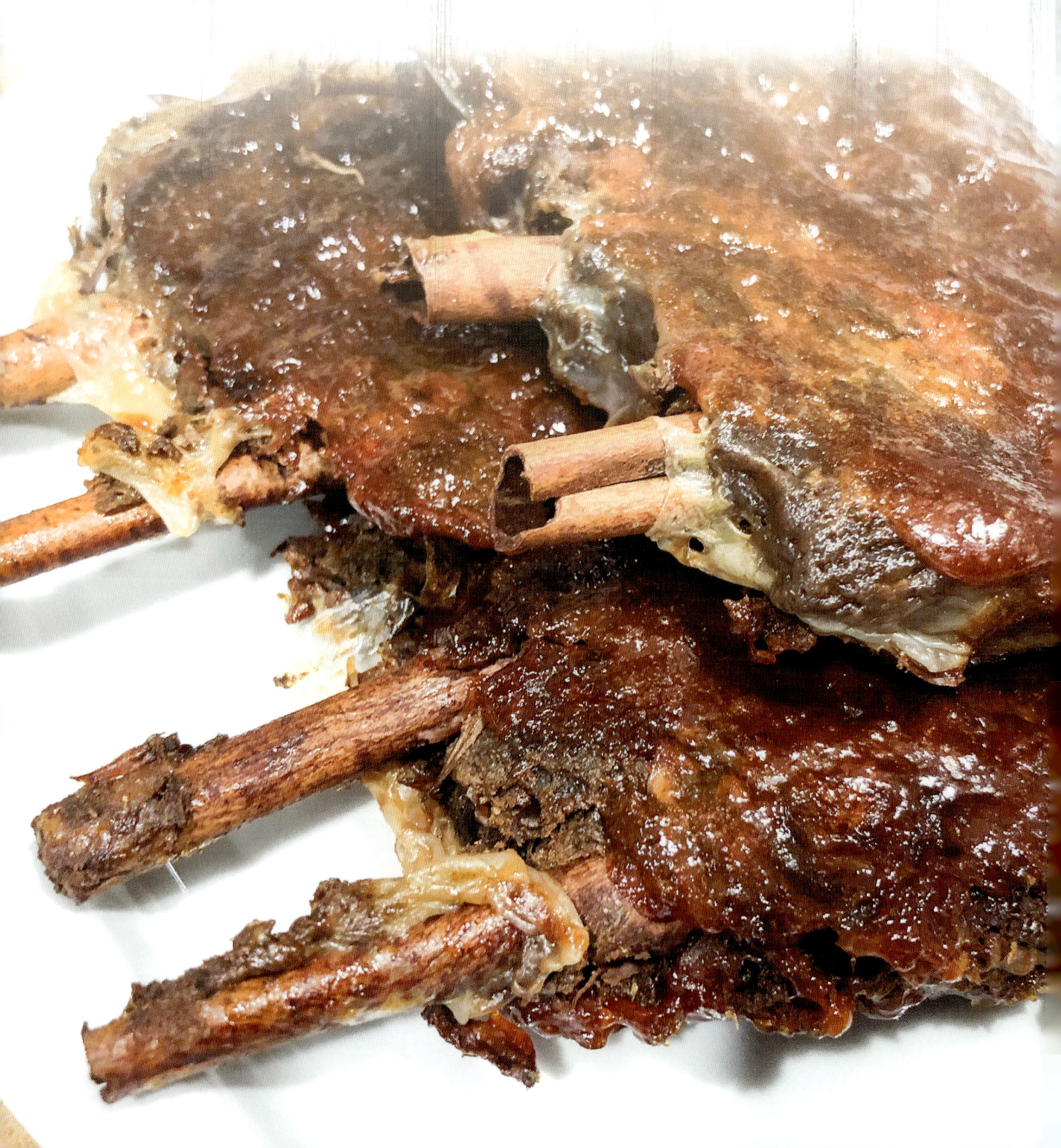

VEGAN RIBS 4.0

I call these my 4.0 Ribs for a couple reasons. It is the fourth time I've transformed my original recipe from 10 years ago. And it's definitely a 4.0 - an A+ recipe. The cinnamon sticks for the ribs is an idea that came to me after a year of contemplating what to use, and then I realized; Cinnamon is in a lot of BBQ recipes, so why not use the stick? It works, and these ARE the best ribs EVER.

YIELD: 4 SERVINGS	PREP TIME: 25 MINUTES	COOKING TIME: 2.5 HOURS

the simple bbq sauce

1 Tbsp liquid smoke
1 cup ketchup
1 cup brown sugar
1/4 cup spicy brown mustard
1/2 tsp salt

the meat ingredients

2 cans jackfruit
1 cup water
1 Tbsp beef-less base
1/2 of the prepared BBQ sauce (above)
1/4 tsp carmel coloring

the dry ingredients

1 3/4 cup Vital wheat gluten flour
1/4 cup almond flour
2 Tbsp tapioca flour
2 Tbsp onion powder
1 Tbsp garlic powder
1 Tbsp chili powder
1 Tbsp smoked paprika
1/2 tsp salt

additional ingredients

4 sheets rice paper - 9 inch square
20 cinnamon sticks

directions

1. Start by boiling the jackfruit in water for 30 minutes. Then drain, and mash up by hand until it has a nice flaky texture. Then squeeze as much juice out of the jackfruit as possible.
2. Make the BBQ sauce by simply combining ingredients and set aside.
3. To make the gluten meat for the ribs you will want to mix the dry ingredients in one bowl and the wet ingredients except for the cooked jack fruit, in another.
4. Then mix the two together, with the jack fruit. Mix well to insure there are no pockets of 'dough' without jack fruit; and that there are no big pockets of only jack fruit.
5. Divide this into 4 equal portions.
6. Now it's going to get messy. You are going to wrap these portions in rice paper. The easy way is to wet a cutting board with water and place a rice paper in the water, then add some more water to the top. You need to soften the paper so we can form it around the ribs.
7. When the paper is softened up a little, place the dough mix on 1/2 of the paper. Make sure to stay away from all sides by at least 1/2 inch, because we need to fold up the sides.
8. Press down the dough on the rice paper with 5 cinnamon sticks inside the meat just like ribs, with a part to grab onto on the outside of the paper.
9. Then you will need to fold up the papers so that it surrounds the ribs and is able to be sealed with the paper on the other side of the rib. Repeat the process with the other three portions.
10. Now that the ribs are encased with rice paper, you will pan-fry them. This will seal up the ribs and give them a great texture. Simply spray the non-stick pan with a little oil spray and sear the ribs on both sides.
11. Place the finished ribs in a baking pan that is lined with parchment paper. Add 1 cup of water to the pan, cover with foil and cook for 1 hour at 350°F.
12. Remove foil, then brush the ribs with some BBQ sauce. Cook for another hour. Every 15 minutes, flip and brush with more BBQ sauce. After one hour they are done. Allow to cool a bit and serve, or chill and reheat when ready to serve.

Chef's Notes

This may seem like a lot of steps, but once you get the hang of it, it is really easy. I would always do a double batch because everyone is going to love these. Watch the video to show you the easy way to knock these out.

Watch the recipe here

VEGAN STEAK SIRLOIN CUT

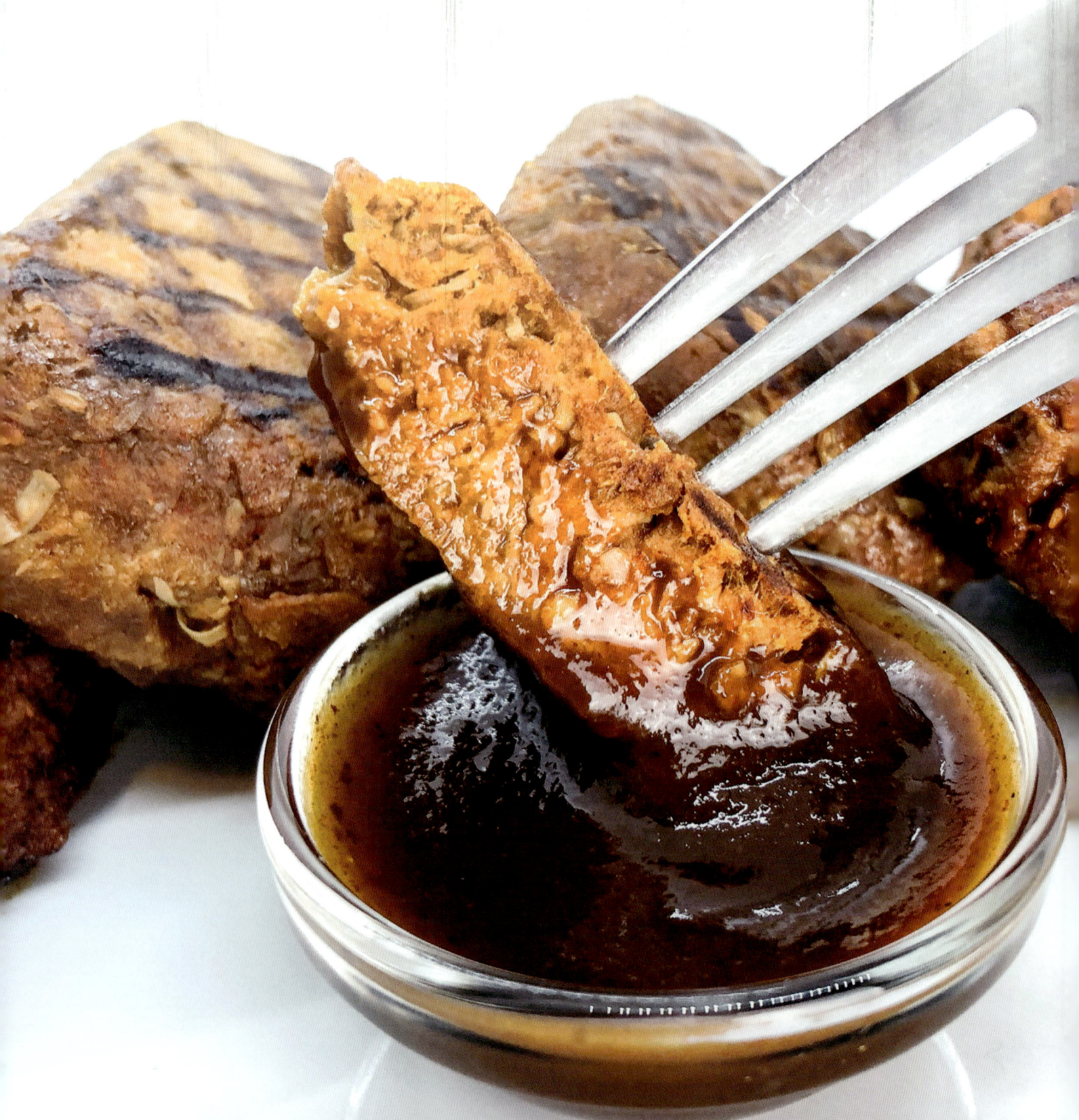

VEGAN STEAK
SIRLOIN CUT

Ding Ding Ding. Congratulations! You just won the jackpot for the best vegan steak ever created. Yes my friends, after a year of testing, the best gluten steak is finally here.

YIELD: 8 SERVINGS	PREP TIME: 20 MINUTES	COOKING TIME: 1.4 HOURS

wet ingredients

3 cans jack fruit (boiled and squeezed)
1 cup canned chickpeas (drained)
1/2 cup water
1/2 cup tomato paste
1/4 cup olive oil
2 Tbsp soy sauce
2 Tbsp beef-less base
1 Tbsp dijon mustard
1 tsp browning sauce
1 tsp liquid smoke

dry ingredients

3 1/2 cups Vital wheat gluten flour
1/4 cup nutritional yeast flakes
1 Tbsp garlic powder
2 Tbsp onion powder
1 tsp cocoa powder
3 Tbsp tapioca starch
3 Tbsp xanthan gum
3 Tbsp methylcellulose
2 Tbsp smoked paprika
2 Tbsp beet powder

marinade ingredients

1/4 cup soy sauce
1/4 cup water
1/4 cup ketchup
1/4 cup A-1 sauce
1 tsp smoked paprika
2 Tbsp brown sugar
1/2 tsp liquid smoke

directions

1. You will first want to boil off the 3 cans of jack fruit in water for 30 minutes. Let cool.
2. Squeeze all the moisture you can out of the jack fruit.
3. In a food processor, blend together all the wet ingredients. You will NOT want to blend extra smooth. Make sure there is some fiber and imperfection to this.
4. In a large mixing bowl, mix the dry ingredients.
5. Add the wet ingredients and mix very well. Begin with a spoon, but you can use your hands to kneed the dough. Kneed it for a good 4 to 5 minutes to make the gluten get some elasticity.
6. Roll it out into a log and slice into 8 steaks.
7. You are going to wrap with foil and put into a steamer for 45 minutes. Fold the foil around the steaks, so as not to disrupt the shape. Don't make the foil wraps too tight. These need a little room to expand.
8. While they are steaming, you will mix the marinade.
9. After steaming for 45 minutes, carefully unwrap and allow to cool. This will help them tighten up before putting the marinade on them.
10. After they are cool, Take a knife and 'trim the steaks'. This is where you give them a true shape of a butchered steak. Don't make them perfect, but you do need to make sure they are level cuts like a steak.
11. Place the steaks into a casserole pan and cover with marinade.
12. Allow to marinate overnight in the fridge, or at least a couple hours, flipping them at least once.
13. They are now ready to finish. You'll want to cook on a lower temperature for longer time. You can fry in a pan, grill on a charbroiler, or even use a panini grill.

Chef's Notes

You can leave it in the marinade for a couple of days. These are great for reheating. And do quite well in the freezer.

Watch the recipe here

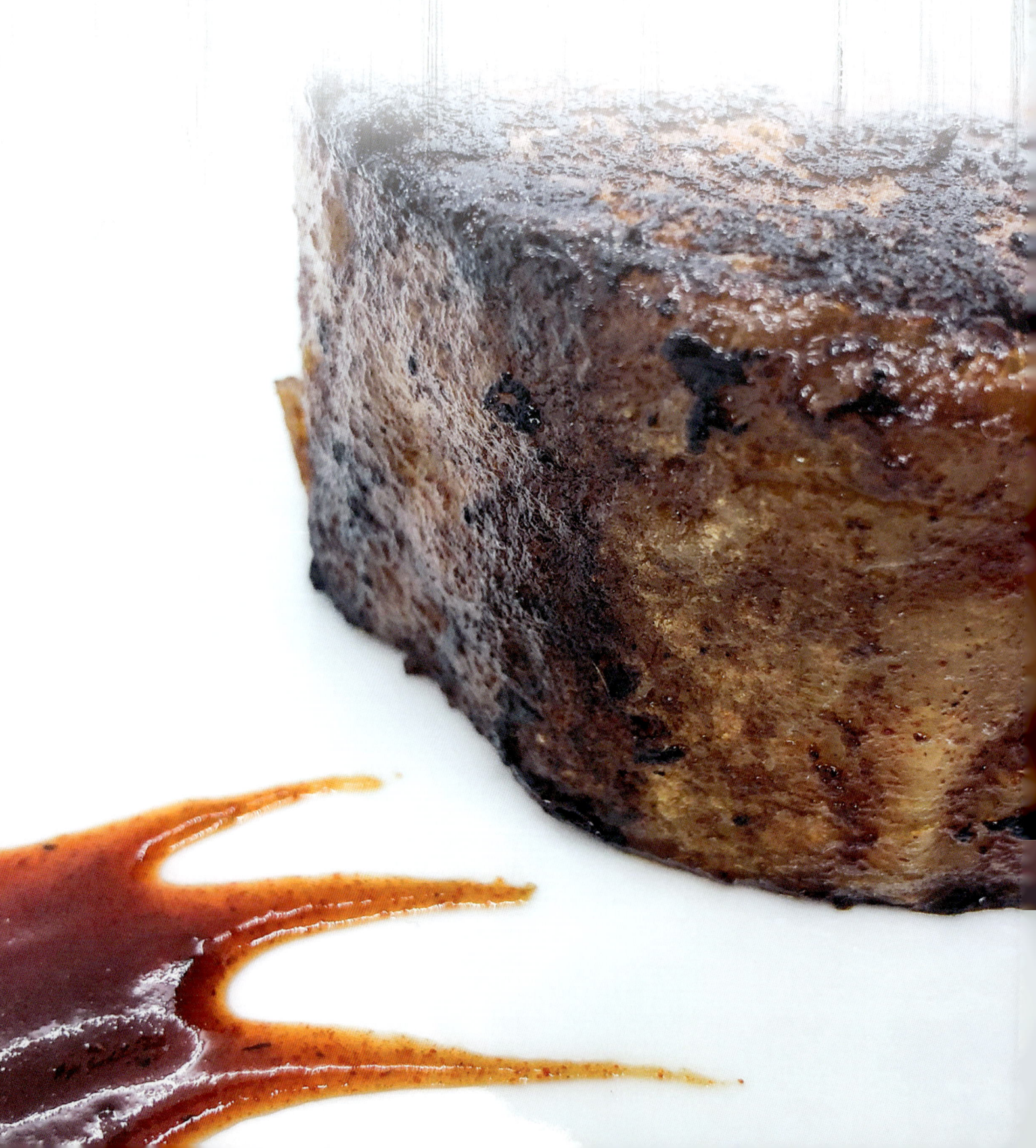

VEGAN STEAK
CENTER CUT FILETS

This vegan steak has the best versatility. You can change the texture, and portion sizes to fit your needs. Simply a great recipe.

YIELD: 6 TO 10 SERVINGS	PREP TIME: 20 MINUTES	COOKING TIME: 1.5 HOURS

wet ingredients

2 cans jack fruit (boiled and squeezed)

1 cup chickpeas (drained)

1/2 cup water

1/2 cup tomato paste

1/2 cup olive oil

2 Tbsp soy sauce

2 Tbsp beef-less base

1 Tbsp dijon mustard

2 tsp browning sauce

1 tsp liquid smoke

1/4 cup nutritional yeast flakes

1 Tbsp garlic powder

2 Tbsp onion powder

2 Tbsp smoked paprika

1 Tbsp beet powder

1 tsp cocoa powder

dry ingredients

2 cups vital wheat gluten

1/4 cup chickpea flour

3 Tbsp tapioca starch

1 Tbsp xanthan gum

2 Tbsp methylcellulose

additional ingredients

6 large sheets rice paper (9 inch square)

for the marinade

1/4 cup soy sauce

1/4 cup ketchup

1/4 cup A-1

1 tsp smoked paprika

2 Tbsp brown sugar

1/4 tsp liquid smoke

directions

1. You will first want to boil off the 2 cans of jack fruit in water for 30 minutes. Then cool.

2. Squeeze all the moisture you can out of the jack fruit.

3. In a food processor, Blend together all the wet ingredients. If you blend smoother, you will have more of a filet mignon texture. If you blend it less, with much more fibers, then it will be more like a NY steak.

4. In a large mixing bowl, mix the dry ingredients.

5. Add the wet ingredients and mix very well. I start with a spoon, but you can use your hands to kneed the dough. Kneed it for a good 4 to 5 minutes to make the gluten get some elasticity.

6. I then roll it out into a log. And then wrap with 6 sheets of rice paper. You will want to lay out the sheets on a wet cutting board, and soften the sheets with water.

7. We are going to tootsie roll wrap the log with parchment paper and foil. Spray the parchment paper with oil spray first, then wrap tight in parchment, and then foil.

8. Steam this for 45 minutes, then allow to cool in the fridge for a couple hours.

9. While they are steaming, I will make the marinade.

10. After the log is cool, I remove the foil wrap, and then I sear the log in a lightly oiled frying pan, on all sides.

11. Cut into pieces. 6 to 8 or even 10, depending what you want to do with them.

12. Place the steaks into a casserole pan where they can get equal marinating.

13. Allow to marinate overnight in the fridge, or at least a couple hours, flipping them when you have the chance.

14. They are now ready to cook. You can fry in a pan, grill on a char-broiler, or even use a panini grill. Just make sure you cook for a longer time on a lower temperature in order to warm throughout. Cooking at lower temperatures for longer time works better.

15. They are done. Yeah.

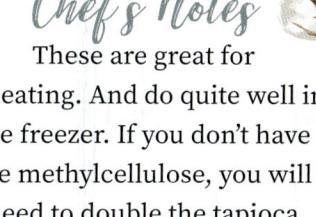

Chef's Notes

These are great for reheating. And do quite well in the freezer. If you don't have the methylcellulose, you will need to double the tapioca starch and xanthan gum.

Watch the recipe here

101